Paul McKenna

'Although I've met many healers over the years, Seka is truly exceptional. She has helped many people all over the world with her amazing ability. She's a remarkable person with a very special gift.'

Greg Rusedski

'Seka has an incredible ability to help the body recover from injury – something I have experienced on several occasions. She also helps me boost my energy during periods of intense performance, making her a key member of my support team.'

Joely Richardson

'Whenever I'm feeling run down or my battery is low, I go to Seka for a boost of energy. I've been seeing her regularly for over four years and I always feel invigorated after a treatment. I recommend her to all my friends, for ailments both large and small. She's a very cool lady.'

Dr Anthony Soyer, MB, BSc.

'I know of no other healer who has the capacity to work constantly at a consistent level and to the same degree of excellence as Seka. I would describe the experience as being given a transfusion of nothing less than love itself.'

Hazel Courteney, Health Journalist of the Year, 1997

'Seka is an extraordinary healer. As a journalist, I have witnessed her healing abilities first-hand, h

and most importantly, also

with seeming incurable

emarkable

YOU CAN HEAL YOURSELF

INCREASE YOUR ENERGY, IMPROVE YOUR HEALTH, BALANCE YOUR LIFE

SEKA NIKOLIC

with Sarah Tay

PAN BOOKS

First published 2006 by Sidgwick & Jackson

First published in paperback 2007 by Pan Books
an imprint of Pan Macmillan Ltd
Pan Macmillan, 20 New Wharf Road, London N1 9RR
Basingstoke and Oxford
Associated companies throughout the world
www.panmacmillan.com

ISBN 978-0-330-44485-9

1 3 5 7 9 8 6 4 2

A CIP catalogue record for this book is available from
the British Library.

Printed and bound in Great Britain by
Mackays of Chatham plc, Chatham, Kent

This book is sold subject to the condition that it shall not,

CONTENTS

FOREWORD

Many years ago I fell down the stairs and twisted my ankle. It swelled up, and the pain was so intense that I couldn't bear to step on it. When I went to see my doctor, he gave me a walking stick and told me that it would be better in a couple of weeks. Later that day I was sitting at home feeling sorry for myself, with my ankle throbbing, when my girlfriend said, 'Maybe I can heal it.' With my scepticism overcome by pain, I told her to have a go. She put her hands on it and closed her eyes in concentration.

It was a few minutes before I realized my ankle wasn't hurting any more. To my amazement, I was able to get up and walk on it immediately. Shortly after, the swelling reduced dramatically. I had become a believer in the power of healing.

A few months later I met Seka Nikolic. I was filming a show about the paranormal: phenomena that we know exist but cannot explain. By that time I had read the scientific studies on the effects of healing. I already knew that it worked, but it had quickly become clear that some people were dramatically better at it than others. It was immediately obvious that Seka's ability was exceptional. I persuaded her to take part in the show and demonstrate her amazing gift, and as a result we became friends.

Energy healing, which is Seka's speciality, is very different to faith healing, which is dependent on the placebo effect and requires the belief of the patient. That difference became remark-ably clear when my father became unwell with rheumatoid arthritis. He was so crippled by it that the doctors told him that it would not be long before he was in a wheelchair. When I mentioned that I'd had a remarkable healer on my show, he dismissed the idea at once because he didn't 'believe in it'. A few weeks later and unbeknown to me, my mother took my father to see Seka. The first I knew of it was when he bounced into my office some days later looking about ten years younger and proclaiming, 'I am healed!'

Since then I have witnessed Seka curing the 'incurable' on numerous occasions. Indeed, we have worked on patients together, combining our efforts to produce amazing results. One of the qualities about her I particularly like is her matter-of-fact attitude towards her incredible skill. If I'd helped someone out of a wheel-chair, I would be so proud I'd want to tell everyone, but for Seka, it's just another day at the office.

This book will give you an insight into one of the most extra-ordinary people I have ever met. It will fire your imagination about what we human beings are capable of. It's worth remembering that at one time nothing was curable – and look how much we can cure now!

Paul McKenna, Ph.D
July 2005

INTRODUCTION

I have been healing for twenty years and during that time I have been asked many questions about my work. When did you start healing? How do you do what you do? What is Bio-Energy? Can anyone heal? Why do I keep getting sick? What can I do to avoid being ill? What's different about your work? Well, I've decided that it's time to answer these questions. I am writing this book to tell you about my gift and my life, to explain what Bio-Energy is and, most importantly, to share with you what I have learned about the power and simplicity of self-healing.

My gift has often been questioned by medical professionals and many of them see a very clear distinction between what they do and the vast spectrum of alternative therapies, but I see a different relationship between Bio-Energy and mainstream medicine. I accept that we need medical practices, and I work very closely with a network of doctors who regularly refer patients to me, so I'm not claiming that Bio-Energy can replace or overrule conventional medicine. What I do believe is that the two fields are complementary and that together they can provide holistic healthcare.

I have always been curious about my gift, and right from the day when I discovered it, I sensed that there had to be a rational scientific explanation of how Bio-Energy works. I looked into the fields of quantum physics and biochemistry and found that the explanations and theories from these disciplines sat more comfortably with me than religious or spiritual ones. But don't worry; this is not a theoretical textbook! I have brought together scientific concepts, esoteric ideas and practical advice to make this book accessible and interesting for everyone.

Whilst I have written about what I do, the focus is not on me or my gift; I hope that my story will put into context how my work has developed and that you will be able to relate to it. What I hope you will find most valuable is the wealth of information on what you can do to improve and maintain your own well-being. You will learn how to become more aware of your energy, which will help you to manage your health and heal yourself. I have included many extensive case studies and a lot of useful advice and tips on how you can improve your health, which you will be able to put into practice straight away.

I have written this book for people who are interested in how the human body works, why we get ill and how we can all achieve extraordinary mental and physical health. This book has the power to expand your beliefs, and whether you are reading this out of professional or personal interest, I hope that it will help you to see new possibilities for the future of healthcare. I believe that we don't know how powerful we are and if we can all tap into our potential, we will become truly healthy, empowered and full of energy. I hope you enjoy what you are about to read.

Best wishes,
Seka

1

MY AWAKENING

I arrived at my office, and the day began as any other ordinary day at work: I got to my desk, checked my messages and started to plough through the list of phone calls and piles of paper. I was very focused when I was at work and was rapidly rising up through the ranks. Mid-morning, my colleague Faroq brought me a document that needed my signature – signing off contracts was one of my responsibilities. I took the paper, scanned it and scrawled my name on the dotted line. But rather than turn back to my desk and continue with my day, I was about to have the most incredible life-changing experience.

Some people say that having a baby turns your world upside down more than anything else, but I've done that and it wasn't that disruptive. Others claim that the death of a loved one will change your life more than any other experience, and that's happened to me too but with comparatively less impact. I suppose people say these things because they measure their experiences against their own personal benchmarks, and those people have never had to face what I was about to.

Faroq suffered from an acute spinal deformity that caused his back to curve very severely. This forced posture limited the movement of his legs and he was confined to a wheelchair. I didn't know Faroq very well, but since I had begun working with him, I had always felt sorry for him. After all, to lose the use of your legs is arguably more life changing than having a baby. I had never thought or felt anything about Faroq that was out of the ordinary, however, so I have no idea why, on that particular day, I chose to help him – and to change the course of both our lives.

As I handed back the contract to Faroq, I was compelled to place my hands on his shoulders. I seemed to be controlled by a force other than that of my rational brain. I wasn't consciously thinking about what I was doing. I was being guided by a deep instinct.

I kept my hands on Faroq's shoulders for about ten minutes. He was becoming hotter and hotter and increasingly alarmed and had started gushing with sweat. It was pretty clear that he was uncomfortable but he wasn't feeling the same pain as me. I was in agony! The pain came through my hands, rose up my arms and shot down my spine, and I was frozen – partly in pain and partly in shock. All I knew was that, whatever I was doing, it hurt like hell. I couldn't take my hands away. There I was with this stabbing pain, completely unable to move. It was as if someone else had taken over my body.

After what seemed like forever I lifted my hands from his shoulders, the pain instantly disappeared from my body, as if someone had flicked a switch. Faroq stood up and looked at me in horror. His look said, 'Who on earth are you?' He was dazed and murmured, 'I can walk. I can walk.' He wasn't shouting with joy, he was mumbling in shock. He turned his back on me, and once he was at a safe distance, he ran out through my office doors, shouting, 'I can walk! I can walk!' The realization had kicked in. There were no words of thanks, just mutterings of horror. I had just had my first healing experience.

It was only a matter of moments before I was engulfed by a mass of people. In those few minutes that I had to myself I struggled to pull myself together. It was as if I'd just had a dream or an out-of-body experience. I was so confused. I was paralysed.

I didn't have a chance to get my head around what had happened before my office was filled with my colleagues, all of whom were looking for a quick fix.

To this day I am still shocked by how they acted: everyone thought only of themselves. They jostled to get to the front of the crowd, and all I could hear was a jumbled list of ailments. 'Seka, my back . . .', 'My arm . . .', 'Over here . . .' By the end of the day, I had treated about twenty of my colleagues. Nobody asked me if I was all right – not one word or gesture of concern. Nobody even asked me what had happened – they all wanted a part of me. From that moment on, life as I knew it was over.

It's so hard to put into words how I felt. I had no idea what I'd done or why I'd done it. I couldn't understand what I'd become. Had I become something or someone else? I wanted to hide from the attention. I wanted to curl up and pretend it wasn't happening. I felt like a freak.

The news spread, and the media were like animals fighting to get my story. Even my closest friends thought of how I could help them rather than how they could support me. I felt alienated from my body and desperately wanted to run away from my power. It hadn't really sunk in that I couldn't escape this – it was a part of me. I couldn't fight it and I couldn't run away. I had no choice but to go with it.

I feel comfortable with things I can understand, and I have always focused on the areas of my life that I could control. Even as a little girl I liked to feel that I had some say over what happened to me and that I was able to change things myself. But this power was something different. It was as if this first incident had to happen like this to show me who was boss: for once, I had no control and I had no choice.

Over the years following this first healing, I did learn how to deal with my gift and how to put it to its best use. I struggled to find out information and to fight prejudice and cynicism along the way. Throughout this journey I learned a great deal about myself and about how Bio-Energy works, and I experienced and witnessed things that I would never have thought possible. I've helped people rid themselves of mental obsessions, I've seen people cured of chronic asthma, and I've helped people bear children when they thought all hope was lost – and that's just a handful of cases.

I realize that this kind of story is the ultimate cliché of an awakening. If you were to dream up a tale of someone discovering that they had healing powers, it probably wouldn't be dissimilar to this. But I'm not going to spin a more elaborate yarn for the sake of drama, because I don't have to. Cliché or not, the reality was dramatic enough.

How Did I Get Here?

I was born in Novi Sad, a large city near Belgrade. There was nothing auspicious about my birth – no full moon, no electric storms and no angels at the bedside. In fact, my whole childhood was pretty normal. I have two older brothers, Brano and Momo, and we have always got on really well. My mother was a teacher, and, although she gave up work after she had children, she was always teaching us things at home. My father was in the Yugoslav army and after he retired, having reached the rank of major, he studied for an economics degree. Given my parents' passion for education, it wasn't surprising that we were encouraged to study hard, and my parents were also great advocates of learning outside of the classroom.

Growing up in a Communist country meant that there was no religion in the strict sense of the word. I went to school with Serbs, Croats and Muslims, and our 'religious' instruction came from the State. My beliefs were shaped by the rules that were dictated by the government and those that were set out by my parents: as far as I was concerned, I had to live within both these laws. It doesn't matter what you call it, any way of living that imposes 'dos and don'ts' becomes your religion.

One of our greatest family interests was astronomy. The stars fascinated me, and at night I would gaze up into the sky from my bedroom window and wonder what other worlds were out there. I couldn't believe that we were the only living things, and I felt insignificant in comparison to the space around me. I was just one little girl in an endless cosmos. I wondered what we looked like from the other planets and imagined we were as small as ants. These musings gave me a sense of perspective, and from an early age I realized that each one of us is just a tiny dot in the universe. It was humbling to look up at the sky, and I soon learned to let go of my ego.

I believed that the stars had immense power. I had three stars that were my favourites, and I would talk to them when I needed reassurance or comfort: I'd ask for help when I was taking exams, and I remember praying to them when a family friend was diagnosed with cancer. When she was given the all clear, I really believed that the stars had worked their magic to cure her.

Either I was born with a caring nature or I learned it from my mother. Even when I was very young, I could sense other people's weaknesses and felt an urge to help them. I befriended those kids who weren't 'cool' and those who had a bum deal: some were too poor to afford new clothes, and some, I knew, lived with alcoholic fathers. I gave time and attention to these vulnerable souls, and I knew my life was charmed in comparison.

My mother was a fabulous cook, and I have vivid memories of our family gathered round the kitchen table. She used to make the most wonderful poppy-seed bread and the fluffiest doughnuts in all shapes and sizes. I can smell them now and I can feel their soothing texture in my mouth. The smell would greet me as I got home from school, and I couldn't wait to wash my hands and get to the table. Whenever I need comfort now, I think back to the sweet smell of yeast and the warmth of the kitchen: the memory feels like a soft blanket.

We moved to Sarajevo when I was two years old, but we had a summer house in the countryside where we would often go at weekends to escape the city. We had such fun there as a family when we were younger, but eventually my brothers and I reached an age when it wasn't the done thing to go away with your parents and we spent more time in the city hanging out with our friends. But my parents loved the tranquillity of the country and would spend weekends there on their own. It was on one such weekend, when I was nineteen, that my parents had a tragic car accident.

They were on their way back home when their car careered off the road, trapping them both inside. My brothers and I were contacted by the hospital and were told that our mother was dead and that our father was in a critical condition. I was in complete shock. The first thing I did was rush to our next-door neighbour's house: Bosa was one of my mother's closest friends. When she saw me turn up in a complete state, she was upset, but she wasn't surprised.

My mother had confided in Bosa the week before that she had foreseen her own death. Being unable to keep it to herself and not wanting to tell any of us, she had told Bosa. I knew that my mother had psychic ability, but she hardly ever talked about it and never really used it, except when she thought there was a real need. She never treated it as a trick to show off with: she didn't agree with things like that. Bosa said that Mum had seen the car accident happen and had known that she'd die but had said that my father would survive. The only thing she hadn't been able to say for sure was when it would happen.

I couldn't begin to imagine what it must have been like for

Mum to know what was coming. I thought back to how she'd been that past week, but nothing unusual came to mind. She had hidden it so well.

When my brothers and I got to the hospital, we were told that Dad had survived. When he'd been brought in, the doctors had thought he was dead, but he'd managed to hold on. His body was completely wrecked: he had a damaged liver, several broken ribs, two punctured lungs, his legs were mangled, and his jaw was shattered. The doctors had little hope that he'd survive. They told us that even if he did live, he'd never be able to walk again.

Mum barely had a scratch or a bruise. When I saw her body, she looked like she was asleep. She looked peaceful, almost serene, but I knew that she was crushed inside: her heart had ruptured and she had died from internal bleeding. The contrast was eerie, but I was relieved that she looked so much like her usual self.

The first few days after the accident were touch and go for my father. On the day that my brothers and I prepared my mother's funeral the hospital called to say that Dad had died. I knew this couldn't be true. I trusted my mother and she would never have said that Dad would live if it weren't true – she wouldn't have given us false hope. We all had incredible faith in Mum, and sure enough, after being proclaimed clinically dead, my father came back to life.

Mum had a very particular presence. She was gentle and strong at the same time, and she exuded wonderful warmth. We weren't alone in missing her. When she died, every wooden object in the house split in half: the wardrobes cracked, a pair of large wooden vases broke in two, and the doors split down the middle. Her power had infused our home, and when she left it, so did her energy.

We kept the news of Mum's death from my father until he was strong enough to take it. He was mentally and physically vulnerable, and losing my Mum would surely have broken him. Whether this was the right or the wrong thing to have done, we knew that the thought of Mum kept Dad fighting for his life.

It was surprisingly easy to hide Mum's death. Dad was confined to his hospital bed, and we told him that Mum was in another hospital, also unable to leave her bed. This kind of situation wasn't unusual in Sarajevo at the time – you were sent where there was room – but we did nearly get found out.

It took us a while to get round to posting Mum's death in the obituaries, and it was so long after the accident that none of the hospital staff made the connection that it was our mother. My father was being transported between hospitals in an ambulance and the nurses with him were reading the paper and commenting amongst themselves that the woman in the obituaries had the same name as one of them 'Look, Zora. Some woman in the obituaries has the same name as you. Fancy that!' The nurses were teasing light-heartedly, not knowing it was my mother's name. The male nurse told me later that my father must have suspected something, as he asked them, 'What's that? Who is it?' They kept the paper from him, but I think he knew what we'd done.

Dad never mentioned the incident to us, not even when we told him the truth. Once he knew she was gone, it would have made no difference to dig up the past. He knew why we'd done what we had and he wasn't angry.

Over the following year and a half my father's face was reconstructed and his organs and bones healed, apart from his left leg. The doctors' prediction that he'd never walk again seemed to be coming true, but neither my father, my brothers nor I could accept it. We had been brought up to stand by our beliefs and to persevere with what we believed in. We steadfastly refused to accept their pessimistic diagnosis: we knew otherwise.

For the eighteen months that Dad was in hospital and for another year after that, I nursed him every day. I would spend all day with him in his hospital room and then go home to cook and clean for my two brothers. I had to take my mother's place to keep the family together, and after each day's chores I would sit down to catch up on my final-year economics lectures for my degree. I wanted to continue with my studies, which had been going very well before the accident. I had been raised to have ambitions and dreams, and I so wanted to work in business. I had the brains, so I just had to find the time. By filling every minute of my day, I busied my mind and distracted myself from thinking about my mum.

Up until this loss, I had had a perfect family life. The only knock I'd really had to take was the death of my grandmother, but a grandparent's death is rarely a great surprise. My mother was only forty when she passed away. I never dreamt I'd be without her so soon. She'd been a great influence over the family and was a very powerful woman. She had incredible charisma and magnetism – to the point of seeming omnipresent.

For the first time in my life I questioned what happens to us after we die. I became more comfortable with the idea of death. I realized that, even though she was gone, Mum was still some-where close to me. I would catch glimpses of her eyes or feel her presence, and her body heat would comfort me when I was lonely or upset. I could tell that it was Mum letting me know that she was close by. Even now I sometimes sense her near me. She's helped me through all my difficult times, and she's guided me as my heal-ing powers have opened up. I loved my mum so much. She had been such a support for all of us, and now that she was gone, I knew I had to look after my family, especially my father.

We All Have Our Limits

I was so distraught after my mother's death that I went into a downward emotional spiral. I was exhausted from dealing with grief and I didn't give myself time to recover. I just kept on going.

One day I collapsed on the street. My body had given up, and it was a warning for me to take care of myself. I was taken to hospital, where I slipped from consciousness.

I remember being in a black room and sensing that there were doors all around me – only one was open. I moved towards the open door and could see a light in the distance. I knew I was close to death, but I wasn't at all scared. I had thought so much about death, and part of me was willing it so that I could be closer to my mum. I felt peaceful and calm, and I made my way through the door and down the dark corridor, away from this life.

I was joined in that dark tunnel by my mother's best friend, Jelena. She looked at me kindly and said, 'Seka, it's not your time.' That was all she said. It was a simple statement, but I knew she was right: I had to think of my father and my brothers, and so I turned back.

When I regained consciousness, I found myself rigged up to a web of breathing apparatus, drips and monitors. I knew I'd been close to death, but nothing seemed out of the ordinary any more. I didn't really know what was happening to me, and the doctors couldn't find anything wrong. I'm convinced that it was delayed shock from my mother's death, but whatever the cause, it was obvious from this incident that I was changing.

My First Significant Healing

When I came out of hospital, all my attention went back to healing my father. One of his legs was gangrenous and the doctors wanted to amputate it, insisting that he'd never be able to use it again. My brothers and I knew that he would get better. We were so sure he'd recover that we signed a disclaimer stating that we took full responsibility for all possible consequences of going against medical advice. We refused the amputation and started to put all our focus on his leg.

I massaged it every day with a blend of herbs and tree sap – a remedy to heal wounds that had been used locally for hundreds of years. I rubbed in the ointment and willed his leg to get better. It started to improve and the gangrene began to clear up. Dad gained strength, and after a few weeks he was able to move his leg. This gave us hope, and we carried on with our own treatment until he was fully recovered.

The doctors were speechless. They couldn't explain it. They tried to fathom out what had happened but they couldn't. I should have guessed then that more was at play: this hadn't just come about because of some massage and a herbal remedy.

My healing powers were really starting to open up. My mother's death had precipitated the awakening of my healing energy. I understand now that all the time I was looking after my father I was healing him. I hadn't yet realized my gift and saw my compulsion to care for him as my duty, but it was as if my power was unleashed when my mother was taken away from me. Years later, after I'd been healing professionally for a while, my brother Momo also discover that he could heal. This must have been our inheritance from our mother. Looking back, it makes sense.

After finishing my economics degree, I wanted to study for a Masters, so that I could one day become a professor. But, first of all, I had to repay the government loan that I'd taken out as an undergraduate, so I got a job in a marketing office. Not knowing then how my life was going to change, I got caught up in the role and started to make my way up the corporate ladder. I had a head for numbers, a gift for languages and a good business degree – all of which positioned me perfectly to work in the strategic-planning department. This was the job I'd wanted, and it also gave me fantastic experience to complement my Masters. I had great ambition, and I worked hard to get what I wanted. My hard work was paying off, and I was pleased with myself. Yet again, I had something to throw myself into.

But it wasn't long before this new-found normality was taken away from me. Something or someone wasn't prepared to let me get on with my life. I wasn't meant to be a businesswoman: I had a different future ahead of me. And so, one momentous day, I was guided down a road from which there was no way back. You already know what happened next and the rest, as they say, is history.

At around this time I became pregnant. I had been warned that the birth wouldn't be easy for me, because the baby was so big, but I didn't realize quite how hard it was going to be. After eleven gruelling hours of labour my contractions stopped. At a loss for what else to do, the doctors and nurses used their elbows, hands and a lot of brute force to pull out my baby. I was in agony and was bleeding profusely, but my baby eventually appeared, with a cheeky lopsided grin. That was all I got to see of my son, Bojan, before the nurses whipped him away to be cleaned up.

The doctors had performed an episiotomy on me to help with the birth, but I found out afterwards that they had cut a main artery in error. As they were checking Bojan, I was bleeding to death. For the second time in my life I was experiencing how fragile my life was.

As I lay there, I felt myself withdraw from the room. I started to look back over my life and was drawn to a memory from when I was six years old. I was playing with my best friend, Vesna. We were making mud cakes in old shoe polish tins and we carefully decorated the cakes with flowers. I felt happy, carefree and very light.

I could see myself in my hospital bed as if I were looking down from the ceiling, and I could hear everything that was being said around me: the nurses chatting, Bojan crying, the clatter of surgical implements and my father's voice. I heard one of the doctors tell my dad that I had died of a thrombosis. I looked on as they lied to hide their careless mistake.

I'd been here before and I knew that death was calling me. I was fearless and kept seeing the smiling face of my newborn son. As I looked down at my tiny baby, I knew that I couldn't leave him. I was married but my husband and I were having some difficulties, and I knew that I was the only person who could really care for my son. I made up my mind to stay for him, and in the moment that I made that decision I re-entered my body. I seemed to be making a habit of shocking doctors!

Same Place, Different World

Within three days of healing Faroq the news had spread across the whole of Sarajevo. People started to recognize me wherever I went. I couldn't walk down the street without people grabbing me and pleading with me to help them, and I couldn't even leave my house without fighting a crowd. Everybody wanted to be healed. I went from leading an ordinary private existence to becoming public property. Some people exalted me as being the Madonna, and some even said that I came from another world, but regardless of who they thought I was, everyone treated me as if I were super-human.

I've told this story so many times, but it still shocks me. In a split second my life had changed at the deepest level. It doesn't compare to anything else – becoming a parent, falling in love, winning the lottery, having a serious accident, losing someone you adore – all of these things rock your world, but they don't make you question who you are. I couldn't rationalize or analyse what I was doing, and it terrified me. I had changed so fundamentally that I was a stranger to those closest to me, and to myself.

I turned to my brother Brano for support. I told him everything that I was feeling and doing and thinking, and I expected him to understand. But how could he understand? If I didn't know what was going on, how could I expect anyone else to? Even my big brother looked horrified. I was so surprised by his reaction, but I know now that he was just in shock. He wanted to help me but he couldn't. He too was afraid of what I'd become.

In desperation, I asked my mother to help me. It was several years after her death but she was my only comfort. I wanted her advice so much. She would have known how to cope. Having had psychic power, Mum was the closest I got to someone who would understand. I suddenly understood why she had kept her gift quiet. I suppose she hardly used it because it must also have been frightening. It made her different, and nobody wants to be around something or someone they don't understand. I could feel Mum's energy and sense her guidance, but I had to face the fact that nothing could bring her back. I was in this on my own. It was the most desperate and desolate period of my life.

At times it felt as if it was all happening to someone else. I no longer felt like myself, and as everything sank in, I grew more and more afraid. I didn't know what to do. I wanted my life to be normal, but for the foreseeable future it was going to be anything but.

I had needed to discover my gift in a dramatic way. It was totally overwhelming and frightening, but it was the only way that I was going to sit up and take notice. Looking back, there were hints over the years that had been too subtle for me to take seriously. As a child I had often fainted when I travelled on the bus, and it was always put down to heat or lack of air, but I now know that I had always been sensitive to energies around me, using my own strength to feed those who were weak. Despite the doctors' shock at my father's recovery, it could be put down to loving care and an old wives' remedy. Neither my brothers nor I ever suspected anything else. Even when I had a sign of my gift, it had meant nothing.

It was the day of my mother's funeral. The house was bustling with relatives and close friends, and my brothers and I were rushing about trying to talk to everyone and make sure they were OK. There was a knock at the door, and Momo went to answer it, expecting it to be more well-wishers. There, on the doorstep, was a stranger, an ordinary-looking woman. Momo waited for her to say who she was, but all she said was, 'Your sister will get your mother's power.'

Momo told me what had happened. Dumbfounded and overwhelmed by the emotion of the day, I put it to the back of my mind and assumed she was a mad woman.

It's funny how we often see what we want to see and hear what we want to hear. Sometimes we pay no attention to things that are thrown at us. The signs were there for a reason, but it was much easier to ignore them than it was to face them. Healing Faroq and the ensuing media frenzy, however, meant that I could no longer ignore the reality of what was happening. Having just got back a semblance of normality after my parents' accident, it was being taken away and I was petrified, but the time had come to face reality, and I just had to get on with it.

In the months following the incident with Faroq, I gradually began to come to terms with my gift. At that time Sunday television in Yugoslavia was full of programmes about lifestyle and life issues, and I regularly appeared on these shows, debating the concept of healing with doctors. I understood so little about my gift, and I often felt overwhelmed at the attention. Cameras. Lights. Probing questions. Aggressive arguments. I had to defend myself and it was exhausting. But the one thing that kept me strong was the knowledge that what I did was real. I may not have been able to explain it, but I could heal. I never thought I'd say that, but my results spoke for themselves.

As my gift developed, my senses became unbelievably strong. It was as if I could feel, hear, smell and see with an astuteness and clarity that I'd never known before. I would pass people on the street and I could hear their thoughts. I couldn't stop myself. I so wanted it to stop. I felt like I was slowly going mad, and I had enough to deal with without hearing about everyone else's problems. This awakening made me realize that I did indeed have psychic power like my mother. It became clearer and stronger as I grew accustomed to my gift, but I decided not to use it professionally. I had a gift to help people relieve themselves of pain, discomfort and disease, not to tell them about their future. It was clear that I had been chosen to work with my power and I wanted to put it to its best use.

Living by Intuition

After the birth I was so engrossed in my work and my son that I had little time to notice how worn out I was feeling. I was treating many people, but I was still unaware of how I was doing it. I healed intuitively and had no idea where my power came from. It switched on when I was treating someone, but what I didn't know at the time was that I needed to switch it off too. Without knowing how to control my energy, it was leaking out of me, and I wouldn't notice until I was totally drained.

I got most drained when I was in crowded places. I would regularly faint on the bus on the way home, as I had when I was a child, but I still couldn't understand why. More than once I passed out in the theatre and put it down to heat and tiredness. It wasn't until several years later that I would understand and eventually learn to manage what was happening to me. This was the kind of thing that nobody could tell me. I was finding out the hard way.

A while after I'd had Bojan I collapsed again. I was pushing myself to extremes once more, and my energy was seeping out of me. I also didn't realize that I had gallstones. My gall bladder had become inflamed, and one day I collapsed on the street in agony and was rushed into hospital – again.

I was wired up to drips and was told I couldn't risk eating or drinking anything other than very weak chamomile tea in case the stones ruptured. I drifted in and out of consciousness because of the pain and the lack of food. But on the third day my deep-rooted will to live took over yet again.

The lady in the bed next to me was pregnant, and her mother had made some pastries for her. They were a bit like Cornish pasties, only smaller, and there was a whole bagful by her bed. I kept looking at them and I could smell them. They smelt so good – buttery, salty and comforting – but I knew that eating anything could put me in serious danger. I lay there for a few moments longer until the sight and delicious aroma got too much. I didn't care. I had to eat.

I heaved myself up off the bed and, with my drip in one hand, grabbed the pastries with the other. I'd been brought up to have impeccable manners, but they all went out of the window. I was taken over by an innate survival instinct. I could barely walk but somehow I still made it to the toilet. I locked the door, sat down and worked my way through what must have been nearly a kilo of pastries. I ate them methodically and mechanically. They were warm, solid and nourishing. It was as if I had never been ill – and as if I'd never seen food before!

Immediately, I felt different. I could feel the energy filling me up, and I was suddenly alert and alive. I was a bit dazed by what I'd just done: again, it was as if I had taken leave of my senses, but it was the right thing because I felt great. I left the toilet and walked back to my bed as if nothing had happened. Nobody would have guessed that five minutes earlier I had been practically unconscious.

I felt completely normal. I apologized profusely to my neighbour, even though I couldn't explain what I'd done. She was too shocked to say anything. The doctors were baffled and refused to let me leave. I insisted that they check me over: I knew that I was fine – I could just tell. They were astounded to find that all of the gallstones had disappeared except for one, which was the size of a grain of rice. They couldn't work out what had happened, but they let me go. They had no reason to keep me in, and I think they also wanted me out of their hospital! Funnily enough, I have never been able to get rid of that one tiny stone. I wonder if, perhaps, it's there to remind me that I'm not invincible.

Proof at Last!

After this incident life carried on as normal – well, as 'normal' as before. My employers were very supportive of me, and given how much of my time at work was spent working on my colleagues, they offered to set up a clinic for me in the office. I treated my colleagues and their families in the day, and in the evening I spent time healing my friends. I was never off duty.

It never crossed my mind to set up my own healing practice, and given the Communist bureaucracy, it would have been impossible anyway. But regardless of the red tape, before I could take this step, I knew I needed to understand more about how I worked. Nobody else understood what I was doing, but they didn't care. They knew that I could help them and that was all they needed to know. But I wanted to know more. I had to understand.

In those days there were no textbooks or 'how to' guides about healing, and so I continued to learn about my powers through trial and error. I wasn't satisfied with healthy people as my sole evidence that my powers worked. I wanted to prove that what I did made scientific sense, so I searched around for someone who could tell me that. I was relatively inexperienced and I needed a boost to my confidence. I thought that external confirmation of my powers would show the cynics that I was a bona fide healer. Maybe then I'd feel normal again and life would settle down.

After searching around, I eventually came across the Scientific Institute for Bio-Energy Research in Milan. The Vatican funded the institute. The Catholic Church was fascinated by those who showed healing ability and wanted to learn more. I contacted the institute straight away, and the researchers there said that they'd be very interested to meet me. I needed to pay my own way to Italy, and luckily, my employers had links with a local airline and were able to help me out with a flight. I set off for Milan, not knowing what to expect.

I ended up staying in Italy for a month. During those four weeks I worked hard with the team of scientists to validate my gift. The scientists tested people of all healing abilities and, based on their findings, clarified what illnesses they were able to heal and what their limitations were. The results of the tests showed that my resistance to electrical currents was six times greater than that of the average person, which means that it's practically impossible for me to receive an electric shock. My ability to produce and conduct electricity was higher than anybody ever tested at the institute. This level of power even exceeded the highest level of certification at the time, so they had to change their certificate to indicate my 'extra supernormal' level of energy.

This information excited the Italian media, and the institute offered me a significant amount of money to stay so they could do more tests. But I didn't want to be a lab rat. I had proof of my gift, which was what I'd gone there for. I'd learned how to work effectively and efficiently, and I was ready to leave Milan, but I wasn't necessarily ready to return home.

When I arrived back in Sarajevo, I had to deal with even more attention than before. The media had a new slant on my story, and they loved the fact that I now had scientific proof of my power.

I had been contacted by a wealthy American businessman, David, who offered to set up a clinic for me in Lanzarote. He invested a lot of money into scientific research in areas that fascinated him and that he thought were worthwhile. He had heard about Bio-Energy and wanted to know more about how I worked. The offer seemed too good to be true. I knew it would be hard for me to carry on living in Sarajevo. I'd had enough of the media attention and wanted the chance to live as normally as possible. It struck me that now that I had been recognized as a healer I could move and set up a new life elsewhere. My marriage, which had been rocky for a while, was on the verge of breaking up, and something deep inside me told me that this was my chance to make a clean break. So I made up my mind to leave Sarajevo, and my family. With my precious son and only a handful of belongings, I left my home.

2

GETTING TO KNOW MYSELF

The Canary Islands are only a couple of thousand miles from Sarajevo, but I felt like I was in another world. I knew that there was no going back, so I decided to look only to what lay ahead of me. I learned early on in life that we can't do much to change what's already happened but we can do a lot to create our future. I threw myself into my new environment and decided to make the most of the opportunity.

David took care of all the administration at the clinic and also gave me a comfortable home and a decent salary. Both my reputation and the clinic's built steadily, and patients came from all over the world – mainland Spain, Italy, Germany, the UK and even from as far afield as America. David funded several scientific research projects and covered the cost of running the clinic. I had a continual stream of patients, and the variety of experience was helping me become more assured. It was the first time since discovering my gift that somebody had showed any genuine concern for my welfare. It was such a luxury to be able to work without having to worry about anything else. All I wanted to do was develop my gift and learn about different cases.

Rather than just be happy with seeing the results, I wanted to know what was actually happening to my patients' bodies as I was treating them and also what was happening to me. For the previous few years it had seemed like my life had been controlled by my power and now I was going to learn how to control it. I wanted to discover all the ways that I could use my energy and see how far I could go. I started to put together what I'd learned in Milan with all of my personal experiences. I felt like I had finally found a sanctuary in which to regenerate and take stock of my new life. I look back now and see that this was a really important transition period for me: away from the pressures of home and the eyes of the press, I grew in experience and self-belief.

Why Does It Hurt?

One thing that had initially confused me was the pain that I felt when I was giving treatments – it seemed to be a major downside to my job! On the day that I healed Faroq, along with general amazement, I remember one of the greatest shocks being the pain. I couldn't understand why I still felt compelled to keep my hands on his shoulders! I knew I had to suffer it, but I had no idea what the pain was or what it meant – all I knew was that I was helping him. Over time, however, I learned that what I feel often mirrors my patient's pain. For example, when I treat someone who is suffering with sciatica, I feel sharp, needle-like sensations from the base of my spine down the sciatic nerve at the side of my leg. It seems that by drawing out the negative energy, I briefly take on the condition, and the pain can be much stronger than my patient actually feels. It's just part of the exchange process – I give them energy and take away their discomfort. My experience isn't always exactly like my patient's. If someone is emotionally out of balance, for example if they're traumatized or depressed, I don't take on their mental state, but I do feel a physical representation of their issue, and with cases like this, it often feels like my hands have been dropped into a pot of boiling water.

When I first started healing, I had no idea how to control this. I would just grin and bear it because I felt so compelled to treat people. It's one of the things I've had to get used to, and over the years I've learned to restrict the pain so that I only feel it in my forearms. I knew I couldn't avoid it completely, so I taught myself to minimize it and mentally rise above it. No matter what condition I'm treating, I am able to block the energy at my elbow and I then shake it off, right out of my own body. As I shake it off, the energy makes a clicking sound, a bit like the crackle of static electricity. I localize the pain rather like pain control in natural childbirth. I don't think many of my patients are actually aware of what I'm going through! This is the most uncomfortable thing for me, but fortunately my pain threshold is pretty high, and if I weren't able to do this, there's no doubt that this energy would wreak havoc on my own health.

Seka and I had just had a meeting and we were heading across London in a cab. I'd had a headache all afternoon and mentioned it to Seka in passing. I wasn't telling her as a hint for treatment, and anyway, I never thought she'd treat me in the back of a moving cab. But as usual she wanted to help.

Seka put her left hand at the back of my head and the other between my eyes. She firmly pressed her fingers into my forehead; it felt so good to have my head cradled in her hands. Despite it being a muggy summer day, her hands were cool. After about a minute she started to extract the negative energy with her right hand by winding it in circles. It looked like she was playing with an invisible piece of chewing gum – so goodness only knows what the cabbie must have thought.

As Seka pulled out the energy, I felt the release in my head. It was instantaneous and a huge relief. Seka, however, was wincing in pain.

She drew her breath in sharply and was pulling an uncomfortable face, but then her pain seemed to subside as she clicked her fingers.

'What does it feel like?' I asked.

'Sharp knives,' she replied bluntly, knowing not to even bother pretending to me that it didn't hurt.

I felt bad – momentarily – but then remembered that Seka experiences pain whenever she treats someone: for her, it's an occupational hazard. Luckily, it didn't last long. I was astounded that the treatment took less than five minutes. We'd barely gone a mile in the Central London traffic and Seka had managed to clear my headache.

Sarah Tay

My Haven

I think back to my time in Lanzarote as a period of peace and stability. I found the energy of the place very comforting and supportive, and I felt safe and relaxed for the first time in years. Having left Sarajevo with nothing but my son and a change of clothes, I spent months rebuilding my confidence and a home, and finally my life was my own. I realized how much I had missed my privacy. I loved being able to do the simplest of things, like going to the beach with Bojan or out for dinner with friends. I did miss my family and close friends, but I didn't regret my decision. I knew that this was a step in the right direction. The island was a haven for me, and I still have very positive associations with it.

Although my patients came from all over the world, there was no need for me to speak any other language. David had provided a very proficient translator, and I managed to pick up some words of English. I didn't know then quite how useful those few words would be. The future seemed only one day long, and I hadn't thought ahead to where Bojan and I would end up. I had no idea that another massive change was upon us.

After I'd been in Lanzarote for a couple of years, I met an English couple – Clive and Elaine Morris. Elaine had been very ill for a while, but nobody could work out what was wrong with her. Her body was very weak, and it was only natural that I offered to treat her. This was the first case of my work to be reported in the British press. *Homes and Gardens* wrote about the Morrises' experience, and Clive told the magazine, 'My wife had been to various doctors. None of them could discover exactly what was wrong with her. She had lost three stone in weight, her hair was falling out, and she was rapidly deteriorating. If we had not met Seka, my wife might not be here today. We have a lot to be grateful for.' After a month of working closely with Elaine, she was free of all the symptoms that she'd been so plagued by. I was thrilled for the Morrises as they could now get on with their lives. I'm very pleased to say that when I last saw Clive a few months ago, Elaine was still very well – over fifteen years since I had treated her.

The Morrises were overjoyed with the results of the treatment. They were so grateful that they suggested that I move to the UK, where they thought my career would have more chance of flourishing. They proposed that we set up a clinic together, and as with David, Clive would look after the business side of things so that I could concentrate on healing. The set-up would be familiar for me, but the environment would be very different. I needed to make a decision.

Bojan is the most cherished possession I have, and every decision I've made since having him has been in his best interests. All of my drive and will to succeed have been so that I could provide anything he needed. At the time he was at an age where his schooling was becoming a great concern for me. My parents had both been great advocates of education, and I had inherited this belief. Although I was no longer using it in my work, my degree meant a lot to me, and I had loved the experience of learning. I knew that there were some excellent schools in London, and I wanted Bojan to have the best opportunities. I made Clive promise that we would find the best school for him, and I also made sure that we'd be able to choose where we lived. With this degree of security and support from the Morrises, I knew I'd be able to learn even more about my work and improve my healing power. As quickly as I'd decided to leave Sarajevo, I decided to say goodbye to Lanzarote. I knew it was time to move on.

A Different Island Experience

When I arrived in England, I set up a clinic with Clive and Elaine in leafy Hampstead Garden Suburbs. The clinic was called The Bio-Energy Clinic, and it had the perfect atmosphere for me to work in. The waiting area was like a living room, and it also had a kitchenette. People could help themselves to drinks and chat with other patients. From the moment people arrived they felt at home, and they would often hang around for quite a while after their treatment. The idea was for them to relax and it worked. I felt safe and as in Lanzarote, I could focus intently on my healing, knowing that everything else was being taken care of.

When I work, I need things to be well organized. The clinic provided the perfect environment and support structure for me, and I had also found a nurturing environment to live in – which, I've since discovered, is quite hard to find in London. As Clive had promised, I found an ideal house in Hampstead. When we went to view it, I knew as soon as I arrived that it was the right house. It felt secure and homely, the area was oriented towards families, and I felt protected from the unfamiliar bustle of Central London. I could get between home and the clinic without having to venture into the unknown chaos of the city, and I really did feel safe and strangely at home. I didn't realize that I was living in one of the most sought-after areas of London but, then again, I've always had good taste!

I have always connected well with people, but it was only when I was in London that people started to keep in touch long after their initial treatment period. Because of the welcoming atmosphere and the high success rate of my treatments, I started to attract a lot of referrals, and as I got to know them better, some of my patients became close friends. It was so lovely to receive bundles of thank-you letters – even though they had to be translated – and it was fantastic, years later, when I could read them on my own. I still have them all. One thing that was mentioned time and time again was the atmosphere at the clinic. Somehow we had managed to create a home from home, for which people were eternally grateful. I know how important simple comforts are when you're unwell, vulnerable, scared and far from the familiarity of home.

I had the good fortune to be introduced to Seka in the spring of 1990. I have a high sensitivity to some drugs and am therefore limited in what I can take, so being introduced to Seka has changed my life dramatically. Before I went for my treatment I had no idea what and who to expect and was slightly scared. But I needn't have been afraid.

Seka and I instantly hit it off – it was as if we recognized each other's energy. My first treatment was for recurrent cystitis, which I had been suffering from for over eight years. Antibiotics helped to a certain degree to alleviate the symptoms, but they never cleared the source of the infection.

The first time Seka gave me healing, the rush of energy that went through my body was so strong that I couldn't stop shivering for a good ten minutes afterwards. Tremendous heat came out of her hands, and she not only unblocked the physical problems of the bladder infection but a whole lot of emotional stuff as well. In that one session I released so many old hurts and pent-up emotions that Seka had to step back a few feet from my energy! It was a very powerful and liberating experience. After the first session I felt very tired – in a good way – and I slept soundly that night.

Seka continued to give me healing for half an hour every day for a week. I felt full of energy and happiness each time she channelled healing. The pain and other symptoms gradually cleared, and after more than eight years of suffering, I haven't had another bladder infection.

M. P. Olinger

It's the Little Things

The language, the place, the people, the roads – all of these things were foreign to me, but the one fundamental thing that I found hard to get used to was the food – it was awful! I say it was awful, but I suppose what I really mean was that it was different. Until then I hadn't realized how much familiarity and comfort we get from food and how strongly we associate it with our home. I was shopping in high-quality supermarkets, so I knew I was buying the best of what was available, but I just couldn't get used to it. The meat seemed a funny texture to me, and the fruit and vegetables lacked the vitality that I was used to. When my father first came to visit, I had to buy ten different kinds of yoghurt before we found one that was close to what we were used to. And then there was the shock of the coffee.

I arrived in London in the days before the explosion of transatlantic coffee shops and European-style cafes, and it was impossible to get a decent hit of caffeine. When I drink coffee, I like a perky espresso, and I couldn't believe that one of the world's major cities was lacking one of life's necessities. The insipid coffee was bad, but the worst thing had to be the bread.

There's nothing quite like the bread back home – fluffy dough peppered with crunchy poppy seeds. My mum baked the most delicious bread, and I remember sitting together as a family to eat her fresh baking – a true home comfort and one that was hard to find here. I'd been in London for nearly nine years before I discovered the Serbian Community Centre in Notting Hill. Eating in the canteen there is the closest thing to being back home, but by the time I'd discovered it I'd got used to English food, and in all my years here I've only been to the centre a couple of times: it's funny how we get used to things.

Over time my friendships grew closer and helped me feel welcome. Bojan settled in at school and also made friends, so it felt as if we finally had a home. I quickly started to make a name for myself, and within nine months of arriving I had a steady stream of patients, many of whom were referred to me by medical professionals who were impressed with my results. I was really getting somewhere.

When my initial three-year contract and business arrangement with the Morrises came to an end, I extended it. I suppose I knew that I was ready to stand on my own two feet, but it was during these last few months working in partnership that I fully grew in confidence. I had spent years developing my skills, nurturing my contacts and getting used to life in London, and I was finally ready to move on and gain more freedom in my work.

Time to Move On

I decided to secure myself a room at the Hale Clinic, near Regent's Park. I was ready to be independent, and the Hale seemed like a good place to position myself. It had, and continues to have, an unrivalled reputation as London's premier complementary health clinic, and it also lured me out of the safety of North London. Being more central than the clinic in Hampstead, it was much more convenient for the growing number of international patients who were coming to see me. The Hale Clinic was more than happy to take me on because of my reputation and my prestigious patient list, and it was during this time that I first started to treat members of the royal family.

The Duchess of York regularly came to me for treatments, but for a long time Prince Andrew remained sceptical about my work. Then he had an unfortunate accident when getting out of his car, which left him with a broken foot. Even after visiting Harley Street doctors, he still had to walk with a stick. Because the Duchess had so much faith in my ability, Prince Andrew agreed to see me, although he was still unconvinced that I could actually help him. I often see people who have this attitude: they don't believe I can help but they also know there's no harm in trying. Andrew's foot was broken in three separate places, but after only three sessions he walked from the clinic free of pain. A royal source told the *Daily Mail*, 'The Duke is the last person you'd expect to choose alternative medicine, but he feels going to the clinic does him the power of good.' For me, one patient is like any other, but results and recommendations like this did help me to build an even greater reputation, and when you're working in a relatively unknown field, referrals are really helpful.

For eight years I was booked up nine months in advance. I worked for six days a week every week and still my waiting list didn't get any shorter. It seemed that alternative therapies weren't quite as 'alternative' as some people believed. It wasn't uncommon to wait up to a year for a first appointment with me, and even now I am often booked up for months in advance. Despite many cynics' views of alternative therapies, it seems that there are a significant number of people who are prepared to take a chance and put their faith in the unknown.

Hitting the Headlines

When I first arrived in the UK in the late 1980s, Bio-Energy was a fairly new practice. The most popular areas of alternative health were acupuncture, reflexology and aromatherapy, so it was no surprise that I had only been in London for a couple of months before I started to attract media interest. After the initial media mania back home I was no stranger to the attention, but the British journalists were less intrusive and the coverage was more manageable. I wasn't mobbed in the street or plagued at home, so I had no complaints. This initial period was the start of a continued strong relationship with the press.

I have appeared in lots of newspapers and magazines, many of which attract very different readers, so I have enjoyed meeting people from all walks of life and from numerous countries. I have always treated the journalists who come to interview me, so that they can experience my work for themselves, and they usually want successful case studies, which is never a problem. I have also appeared on several radio and television programmes. This initially seemed like a good way to boost my profile, but I was badly bitten. I agreed to appear on a popular morning chat show, and not knowing much about the programme, I was shocked when I couldn't get a word in edgeways: rather than an open discussion, the show turned into an uncontrollable free-for-all. I found it totally draining and swore never to do that kind of television again. The shows I've most enjoyed taking part in are the ones that show me at work, rather than those that want to pick an argument.

I also started to attract interest from medical professionals who were impressed with how much I helped their patients. The belief and support of the medical profession is an accolade that many alternative practitioners only ever dream of, and I had begun to achieve it within a short while of practising in the UK. The number of doctors who regularly and readily refer their patients to me has grown steadily, and I also make referrals back to them where necessary. I believe it's most beneficial to the patient when we work together.

The Control Issue

During my first few years away from Sarajevo I had learned a lot about my gift. I still can't get over how much I had to take on board. There were no manuals or guides on Bio-Energy – I just had to learn through experience – and some things took more time to sink in than others. One thing I hadn't paid much attention to was the impact that my work was having on my own health. I knew how to deal with the pain but my own energy was soon to become a big issue: it was slowly draining away and I didn't realize it.

Every time we connect to another person, physically or mentally, we exchange energy. Do you ever notice how you feel after spending time with another person? You may find that some people make you feel energized and positive, whereas others drain you of all good feelings. All you have to do is think of a time when you were with a depressed person and remember how you felt afterwards: you probably felt very low or tired. Then think of a time you spent with someone fun and uplifting: I bet you came away feeling recharged and invigorated. The people we spend our time with have a very real effect on our energy levels. We can't see the interaction of energies but we know it happens.

People who work in caring industries, like doctors, nurses and alternative therapists, are particularly at risk of becoming drained. They are continually in contact with a whole mix of energies, and if they are to maintain their own well-being, they have to learn how to conserve their own energy by staying emotionally detached from whoever they work with.

Because Bio-Energy treatments affect patients very deeply, the energetic connection I have with them is profound – that's how I can heal them. It's as if I plug them into my own energetic grid whilst I pass on energy. It took me a long time to realize that I could become drained if I didn't take care. I know now that I can work without harming myself, but for years my body was giving me warning signs and I didn't read them.

Just like in Sarajevo, I found myself getting tired and weak. I had been putting in twelve-hour days for six days a week, and it was becoming harder for me to keep up my own energy levels. I thought I was just overworked. I was treating patients very intensely and this was taking its toll. It was my job to help other people, and I always put their needs first – whether it was friends, family or my patients. I was overlooking my own well-being partly because I just assumed my health was strong and partly because my awareness of energy hadn't completely developed. I could treat people intuitively, but I hadn't grasped total understanding of how profoundly my energy was being affected. As with any great gift or power, it's sometimes hard to keep a check on it – and from time to time I was surprised by how low I could get.

I was still experiencing the extreme fatigue I'd felt all my life when I went to crowded public places, like the theatre or cinema, and would often be close to collapsing by the time I got home, but I still couldn't understand why. It felt as if someone had sucked the life out of me. I know that crowds can be tiring, but my reaction was a bit extreme. It was then that I came to learn that this was happening because my energy channels were wide open. When there were lots of people around me, they weren't consciously 'stealing' my energy but, as if by osmosis, those people who needed a boost, or who were ill, would attract my energy because

I had left myself vulnerable. My energy was drawn to them like iron filings to a magnet because I hadn't learned to switch it off. I was a sitting target. I had to learn to protect myself so that I could lead a normal life. I got into the routine of closing down my energy channels, like turning off a tap, so that I kept some energy for me. I find it hard to explain how I do this because it's something I do automatically, so the best way to explain it is by telling you what I do on a practical level: as soon as I have finished treating people for the day, I think about all of the mundane things I have to do, like cooking, shopping and cleaning! By switching my attention to everyday tasks, my energy closes down from being in the healing state to being in a state where I can function in the 'real world'. Regardless of the fact that I'm a healer, I have chosen to live in one of the world's busiest and most densely populated cities, and I have to protect myself accordingly so I don't have to be a recluse.

Although I now close down my channels automatically, I still avoid situations that I know will drain me. When I can't, I have to make sure that I control my energy with my intention: this was the key thing I had to learn. I have to decide not to become emotionally involved with my patient, and I tell myself to stay detached. When I first started to heal, I thought I could only work well if I was emotionally attached, but now I know that to be really effective, I have to be as strong as I can – and that means staying above all emotion. That may sound cold, but it enables me to do the best job possible. It's because of this that I find it hard to treat those closest to me. Learning that I wasn't invincible was a very valuable lesson. I now protect myself out of habit and don't even need to think about it. I rarely get crashes any more. Whilst it was distressing to get slumps in the early days, there were also times when I was caught unawares by my sudden bursts of energy.

One day I was arriving home from work and was just closing the front gate behind me when, out of the corner of my eye, I spotted a gang of teenage boys over the road. They were trying to break into a neighbour's house. My first reaction was to try to get their attention, to let them know I'd seen them. I waved my arms and called to them and one of them promptly turned and gave me the finger. Instinctively, I felt anger rise up inside me like a boiling geyser. You hear stories of people harnessing supernatural strength when they have to; well, I found myself hurdling my garden gate and before I could rationalize what I was doing, I had lifted up a couple of the boys into the air. My physical outburst was overwhelming, but what came out of my mouth was even scarier! They saw that I meant business and they scuttled off. I was shocked by my own power – it seemed to have come from an emergency reserve. I had no idea how strong I could be.

Knowing My Boundaries

To keep myself balanced, I tried to take regular holidays, but for a few years I was completely focused on working and saving money, so it was hard to schedule a break. When I did go on holiday, I would return to Lanzarote. It was familiar and I found it very relaxing, but it wasn't always easy for me to switch off. On one holiday I was lying on the beach when I heard a woman screaming in agony. As anyone in a caring profession will tell you, even when you're supposedly off duty, you can't switch off if you know you can help. This lady had been jumping waves when she landed badly and broke her shoulder. She had made it back to the shore and was clearly in need of medical attention. I automatically ran over and placed my hands on her shoulder until the ambulance arrived. The pain subsided dramatically, and I kept my hands on her all the way to the emergency department. The ambulance crew couldn't believe how little pain she was in – little did they know that I was in agony!

Over time I did learn to take time out for myself to recharge. I began to explore my new home, but there are still so many things I've yet to see in London and the rest of the UK. I couldn't have continued at the same frenetic pace, and I knew that to be the best Bio-Energy practitioner, I had to put my own health at the top of my priorities: if I wasn't well, I was no use to anyone else.

My move to the Hale Clinic had proved to be the right decision, but after a while I chose to work there just for the mornings and took a room at the Kailash Centre of Oriental Medicine in St John's Wood in the afternoons. It felt good to be in control, and this new independence also made me feel more at home. My home life was stable, and Bojan was happily settled too. After leaving school, he decided to go to music college to pursue his passion. Although I've never lost my accent, my English was becoming a lot better and I no longer needed the translator that I had initially relied on. London had become home and I was holding my own. I didn't need to rely on anyone else – and it felt great.

3

THE SCIENCE OF BIO-ENERGY

I managed to get comfortable with the practical side of my gift through trial and error, but as I mentioned earlier, I only really started to piece together a scientific picture of my power when I was at the Institute for Bio-Energy Research in Milan. I wanted to learn about the science behind my gift so I could understand more deeply how I affected people. I was probed and prodded and wired up to countless devices, and my hands were submitted to extremes of temperature and electric currents. These experiments finally confirmed what I had suspected for a while – that my energy was a bit like electricity.

When we think of electricity, we tend to picture machines, pylons and power stations, but what we often don't think about is that the human body is a machine driven by subtle electric currents. Have you ever touched someone and felt an electric shock? It's a very real sign that our bodies are full of electromagnetic energy, and it is this energy that I use for healing.

The Electromagnetic Body

We need electromagnetic energy to function properly. The brain, the body's headquarters, is made up of more than 100 billion nerve cells and the brain sends commands through these nerve cells, by electric pulse. The body's nervous system then sends messages via electrochemical impulses, and it is these signals that allow us to breathe, move, talk and do all of the things we take for granted.

Some of the most well-known research on electromagnetic energy was done by Dr Harold Saxton Burr, a neuroanatomist at Yale University. He used a conventional voltmeter to measure changes in the energy field of plants, animals and humans, and he found that diseases like cancer caused significant changes in the electromagnetic field of living organisms.[1] With information like this filtering into the medical community, it is now considered normal to use energy to treat illness – some examples being radiation therapy for cancer, electromagnetic fields to heal bone fractures and electricity to control pain.[2] On a more familiar level, most people have seen television dramas or films in which someone is hooked up to an electrocardiogram (ECG) machine. This is attached to a monitor that shows the electrical activity in the heart. When someone passes away, they are said to 'flat line' because the monitor reading shows that electrical activity in the heart has ceased. So you can see that electromagnetic energy plays a vital role in our well-being.

How does this relate specifically to healing? Well, the brain communicates with the immune system by electrochemical impulses, so the body can only heal itself when it has sufficient energy. So Bio-Energy works on the premise that we need strong energy to maintain our health or heal ourselves. When our energy circulates freely, we can regenerate quickly and effectively, but when our energy is weak or blocked our health suffers.

In Milan the scientists ran all sorts of tests on me to see how strong my energy was. From what they already knew about heal-

1 Dr Harold S. Burr, *The Fields of Life: Our Links to the Universe* (New York, 1972).
2 Richard Gerber, MD, *Vibrational Medicine: New Choices for Healing Ourselves* (New York 1988).

ing energy, this then clarified that I really could work with people. They used instruments to measure my ability to conduct and resist electrical currents and also tracked the temperature of my hands during treatments to prove that the heat I gave off was due to healing energy and not because of changes in my body or the ambient temperature. As I said earlier on in this book, the scientists found that I had an unprecedented level of conductivity, which means that I can feed very powerful energy into my patients at consistently high levels, and they had yet to see human energy work in this way.

These tests were the external confirmation of my gift. I had known from the start that something incredible was happening inside me. I could feel that it was a truly physical phenomenon, one that seemed beyond my control, and my results with people were so rapid and dramatic that it was clear that I was changing people at a deep, cellular level. With this information, I had a clearer idea of what I was doing.

By holding my hands above the body, I can sense how someone's energy is moving. I know which organs or cells are imbalanced, and I know where there is an excess, shortage or blockage of energy. It's as if I'm reading their medical history with my hands. I then use my own energy to retune their levels to the correct frequency and return them to a healthy state. I often think of myself as a transformer: just as transformers step up or step down voltage, I instinctively increase or decrease the energy that I need to channel in order to bring someone back to the correct level. I don't consciously do this – it's something I do intuitively, which is why it's a gift. But whilst very few people are able to sense as acutely as me, we are all able to sense energy to some degree, and by realizing your own sensitivity, you'll hopefully gain a better understanding of what I do.

The Human Frequency

Have you ever met someone and felt an instant connection with them? You can't explain it: it's not necessarily because of physical attraction – it's just that you're on the same wavelength. Well, believe it or not, this feeling of attraction is because of our energy. I bet you've heard the phrase 'magnetic attraction', but I wonder if you know quite how accurate it is.

Because of the flow of electric energy in our body, each of us is surrounded by our own electromagnetic field. This may sound a bit strange, but remember that we live inside the greatest electromagnetic energy field, the Earth's gravity field. We take it for granted but without it we'd be flying around in space. It's such a vital part of our existence that we don't give it any thought. Well, the gravity field is not the only electromagnetic field that affects us. We live in a web of energy fields. On a micro level each and every thing in the universe has its own energetic pull, and that's what we feel when we connect with someone. Our magnetic field gets close to theirs and we attract each other. But energy fields don't always attract one another. Like magnets, we can also be repelled by each other. I bet you can think of someone with whom you clash. With attraction, you can't always explain why but you just don't feel comfortable around them. Energy fields interact in different ways, and these feelings are due to the energy inside us. I like to refer to this energy as the human frequency.

To take a slightly different look at the human energy field, let's turn to something that is a bit more familiar – the radio. Every radio station has its own frequency, so you know what frequency to tune in to if you want to listen to a particular station. The energy that is generated by our own electromagnetic field vibrates in a similar way to a radio wave, so we too have a personal frequency that distinguishes us from other people.[3]

Our own personal frequency is like our home station. For the sake of illustration let's say that I have a frequency of 92.3 FM and you have a frequency of 104.1 FM. Just like we have our own phone number, passport number and unique DNA fingerprint, we have our energetic frequency. In reality, we can't label human frequencies by using numbers; we can only tell when a frequency feels right by paying attention to what our instinct tells us.

So how does this tie in to Bio-Energy? Well, when we're tuned in to our own vibration – the set frequency that we're born with – we feel healthy and strong, but this frequency can change. Just as a radio signal becomes crackly when it experiences interference from other channels, our body's frequency can also be disturbed by frequencies from other people, places, sounds and even thoughts.[4] When our energy is weakened or when it shifts from its equilibrium, the vibration changes, and this shift is reflected by negative symptoms in the body's chemistry, structure and function.

To go back to the example I gave earlier, say that your natural healthy frequency is 104.1 FM, but when you get run down, your energy shifts and your frequency changes to 102.6 FM; by being out of sync with your natural vibration, your immunity is weakened, you feel under the weather, and you experience symptoms such as a runny nose, sore throat and heavy limbs. By resting, eating well and drinking plenty of water, you can return your frequency to normal and you feel well again. Bio-Energy is about directing and feeding the body's energy in order to achieve the correct frequency and therefore the best state of health possible. An illness like the common cold happens when your frequency falters,

3 Michael and Eva Nudel, Ph.D, *Health by Bio-Energy and Mind* (New York, 2000).
4 Toni Bunnell, Ph.D, 'A Tentative Mechanism for Healing', *Positive Health*, issue 23, December 1997.

which isn't too serious, but people tend to come to me when their energy has gone much further off track.

Whilst we can often correct our own frequency, most people lack awareness of their energy pattern. We so often miss the subtle warning signs and only realize we're unwell when the symptoms are more tangible – we're in pain, we feel weak, we're exhausted, our skin flares up, we put on weight and so on. It's like walking a tightrope: if we're just beginning to wobble, we can get our balance back, but if we start to wobble and don't correct ourselves in time, we fall. Most people only pay attention to their health when they've fallen – and that's when it's harder to get balanced again. It's at times like these that I can help. Because of my gift I can retune other people's energy systems and energy fields so that they return to a state of equilibrium and health. I am able to influence a frequency much more quickly and effectively than if someone were correcting it themselves, and then once they are back at their correct frequency, they can rid themselves of disease.

It was early January and I had started to get aches in my joints and muscles. The pain began in my feet, which were very tender, and it was painful to walk. My fingers felt very swollen, although they didn't look it, and it was difficult to bend them and do things with them – they felt numb. There were no other physical signs, but the only way I can describe the feeling is that my body felt as if I had been poisoned. I was also incredibly tired; I had no energy at all and slept through most of January.

I went to my doctor for blood tests, but they all came back negative. Although I was in so much pain, with negative blood tests and no physical symptoms, my doctor seemed at a loss as to what to do with me.

I heard about Seka through my boyfriend. He had been to see her and had marvelled at the wonders she performed. So I decided to see her for an initial consultation.

Seka told me in the first session that she felt the pains were coming from the top of my back. I thought about it and realized that before the pains had got bad, I had had a very stiff neck and aches in my shoulders – this hadn't crossed my mind before. Maybe this was the root of it.

I left that first session with more energy than I had had in a month, so I booked a course of 5 sessions. In the second session I vividly remember feeling as if my whole body was floating. Seka was holding my head, and it felt as if the rest of my body was floating freely above the couch. I could feel energy flowing up my legs as Seka worked on my feet, and when I left after the second day, I could walk down the stairs freely – no more hobbling down one step at a time! Every day I had more and more energy. The biggest change was after the fourth session, when I left feeling like my old self, with energy to go out and do things once again.

It was a relief to know that whatever I had was treatable, I didn't have a scary debilitating disease, as some people had kindly pointed out I may have! Since then I have been improving more and more. I have had some bad days but also days when I feel healthy. When I look back, there have been big improvements each week.

It was great to meet Seka, and my treatments have brought relief to both my physical and mental well-being. My thanks to Seka, and I will continue seeing her to maintain this well-being until I am fully back on form.

Lucinda

The Positive Side of the Negative

To me, it seems clear that science can explain how Bio-Energy works, but this isn't a widespread opinion. Some scientists refuse to accept that healing can occur through positive energetic change, but ironically, they do accept that illness can be caused by negative energy changes.

There is increasing awareness of the dangers of long-term exposure to certain electromagnetic fields – like those given off by microwaves, mobile phones and pylons – and there is now clear evidence to show that they can cause certain diseases. Some studies suggest that conditions such as leukaemia, brain tumours, abnormal pregnancies and ME are due to extensive exposure to electromagnetic pollution and radiation. Because of these claims, the UK's independent Health Protection Agency has a department, the Radiation Protection Division, which is responsible for researching how these forces interact with the human body.

Though unfortunate and potentially damaging to health, in my eyes this 'negative' evidence helps to cement the argument for Bio-Energy: if the body's balance can supposedly be disturbed by forces that affect its natural electricity, and therefore its health, then it makes sense that the reverse is also true – that energetic balance can be restored in the human body by the force of positive electromagnetic fields. So why is it so hard to accept that the positive use of similar fields can bring about improved health? Luckily, there is some very solid scientific theory to back up my argument.

Albert Einstein is thought by many people to be the most important physicist of the twentieth century. He is best known for his theory of relativity, and one of the offshoots of this theory is the concept that energy and mass are interchangeable. In this theory he claimed that whether something is tangible (like our physical body) or whether it's intangible (like our energetic frequency), it's all made of the same universal substance: solid, liquid or gas. Quite simply, everything is made of energy.

If this theory holds true, then it gives us an excellent basis for understanding Bio-Energy. Just as ice, water and vapour are all made of H_2O, our physical body is made of the same substance as our energy. Conventional doctors work on the physical body, and

I work on the energetic body. Because these are essentially the same, we are both able to affect the physiology of the body, but we do so in different ways.

Unfortunately, there is some resistance to the concept of Bio-Energy healing, and this resistance makes it hard for Bio-Energy practitioners to involve scientists in validity studies. My work can't be cut open, viewed under a microscope and monitored, and many scientists don't believe in things that they can't see, measure or collect in a test tube: to accept that such powerful energies exist would mean shaking the foundations of their beliefs and profession. The view of Bio-Energy is gradually changing as more people accept that healing and other complementary health methods should be scientifically researched. There are, however, already centuries of evidence.

The Old Timers

When I first started to research historical evidence of Bio-Energy, I was amazed by how much I could find. One of the earliest records of Bio-Energy was in the early sixteenth century. Swiss physician Philippus Aureolus Paracelsus argued that there was a substance that filled the entire universe. He said that it linked everything and everyone, and he also claimed that his invisible substance had magnetic and healing properties. He also believed that certain people could harness this energy to heal others.[5] Doesn't it sound like he had discovered Bio-Energy?

In 1778 Franz Anton Mesmer, who is known as being the father of modern hypnotism, claimed that all humans had an electromagnetic field around their body, which he suspected could interact with and influence that of other people. He also said that

5 Richard Gerber, MD, *Vibrational Medicine: New Choices for Healing Ourselves* (New York 1988).

he could heal using fluidum, a substance that filled the universe and that connected all living things.[6]

Michael Faraday, the great British chemist and physicist, worked with another scientist, James Clerk Maxwell, to come up with field theory. This theory stated that each magnetic field has a force that can interact and disturb other fields around it. Similarly, Dr Liebault, a nineteenth-century French doctor, believed that a human energy field could have an energizing or draining effect on that of another.[7] It all sounds a bit familiar, doesn't it?

In the twentieth century, knowledge about human energy started to increase. Dr Robert Becker, of Upstate Medical School, put together a map of the body's complex electrical field, which he claimed changed shape and strength when the body underwent physiological and psychological changes.[8] This is something that I can sense when I treat someone, so to discover that a doctor had recognized this in the 1960s was comforting for me. Maybe I'm not mad, after all.

A more recent study, undertaken by the Annie Appleseed Project, a non-profit-making organization, was presented at the Eighth International Congress of the American Academy of Anti-aging Medicine in Las Vegas. It showed that chronic wounds treated with very low electrical currents heal more quickly than they do with standard treatments. One of the doctors involved in the study, Dr Alfred J. Koonin, said, 'We don't completely understand why it works. What we do understand is that the device seems to act as an ultra-powerful antioxidant that knocks out infection, stimulates blood flow and encourages cell regeneration. In layman's terms, it takes an electrical system that's out of whack and sort of normal-

6 Gloria Alvino, 'The Human Energy Field in Relation to Science, Consciousness and Health' (1996).
7 *Ibid.*
8 *Ibid.*

izes it.'[9] This too sounds to me like evidence of Bio-Energy in action.

In the last few decades scientists have gone from being adamant that there was no energy field around the human body to being certain that there is, so who knows what will happen over the next few years. I encourage more research because I feel that it would open up the field of healing to a wider audience. My confidence doesn't come from a place of arrogance. To me, my ability is a fundamental part of who I am and it can be explained in common-sense terms. I also know that further research into Bio-Energy would bring our healthcare system one step nearer to being fully holistic.

Bio-Energy – Not a New Phenomenon

Whilst the West is at the forefront of many scientific and medical developments, it is only just coming round to the same ideas about human energy that the East has been following for centuries. There is some evidence that the concepts underlying Bio-Energy originated in China about 5,000 years ago. The Eastern model of health is based on the principle of 'chi', or 'qi': chi is the vital energy force that nourishes the body, and the Chinese believe it to be more important to life than food, water or air. Chi is said to flow around the body in meridians, or energetic pathways, and this flow of chi needs to be in balance for the body to be in good health.

Hindus have also founded their health practices on this energy, which they call 'prana'. They believe in the concept of energy centres, known as 'chakras'. Chakra is the Sanskrit word for 'wheel', and these energy centres are believed to be whirling vortices of energy. The seven major chakras, each of which is supposedly

9 For more information, visit www.annieappleseedproject.org.

linked to a major nerve plexus or endocrine gland, are spread roughly along the midline of the body: at the top of the head, known as the crown chakra; at the third eye, which is in the centre of the forehead; and around our throat, heart, solar plexus, abdomen and the base of the spine. These wheels of energy are said to suck in energy from the external forces in the universe, which they then transform to a level that the body can cope with so as to nourish and energize.

The concept of complementary and energetic medicine has also been around for many centuries in Eastern Europe. I grew up very familiar and comfortable with the idea of alternative healthcare. We had free healthcare, but we didn't use it: with herbal remedies and a daily dose of live yoghurt to boost the immune system, we managed to keep very well. People used herbs for everything from stomachaches and kidney problems to headaches. As I mentioned in Chapter One, Even when my father's leg was gangrenous, we used an old herbal remedy to help clear up the infection. It wasn't seen as 'weird' or 'freaky' but as a normal thing to do. It was common to visit a herbalist, who would make up a 'melum' – a miracle cream with a secret recipe – and these herbalists are as respected as conventional doctors for their knowledge and skill.

In our biology lessons at school we learned about anatomy and physiology, just like children in other countries, but we also learned about herbalism. Even in our home economics classes, alongside cooking, table manners and housekeeping, we learned how to prepare herbs. Once a month our teacher took us into the local woods. We were taught how to recognize the various plants by their shape, smell and where they grew. On a recent visit back home I was pleased to see a group of schoolchildren being taught the same things. These old traditions have lasted because they are part of the culture – and also because they work!

One of the countries most open to these concepts is Russia. At the Institute of Radio Engineering and Electronics in Moscow, Professor Yuri Gulvaev has achieved a 98 per cent success rate when using electromagnetic therapy to help treat psoriasis. The Russian Ministry of Health has also approved a device called the YAV-1. This machine uses extremely high-frequency radio waves to treat ulcers. Doctors, who have used this machine on 7,000 patients suffering with ulcers, have managed to achieve a 91.7 per cent healing rate.[10] Developments like these prove that external electromagnetic fields can affect the body's biological functions, but it doesn't automatically follow that all medical professionals are open to accepting this concept. Throughout my career I have come across doctors who are very closed in their views, and I have also come across some who are intuitive and holistic.

One of my close friends and long-standing patients, Dr Anthony Soyer, has been referring patients to me for fifteen years – ever since he was recommended to me. He has spent many years in China studying martial arts and alternative health practices and so has been interested in complementary health for a long time. He fuses his medical training with his knowledge of the complementary to seek an understanding of what I do.

> I met Seka through a friend of mine, Maya. Seka had not been in London for long, and she was still practising in North London. At the time I was *TV-am*'s medical researcher and I was looking into healing and cutting-edge therapies, so I was particularly fascinated by Seka's work.
>
> Several years later I had an injury to my wrist from martial arts training. This was soft-tissue trauma from a heavy impact to the tendons and nerves, and it led to a progressive and complete loss of grip in my left hand. I used a number of treatment modalities, including compression bandages, homeopathy with arnica tablets and cream, Rhus.

10 Alfred Riggs, 'The Association of Earth Radiation and Other Fields with Specific Diseases', *Namaste*, vol. 6, issue 4.

Toxicodendron, high-dose Vitamin C, magnetic therapy, osteopathy and old-fashioned rest, but to no avail. Nothing worked, and I couldn't even grip cutlery properly. After six weeks of suffering and continuing decline I decided to see Seka.

During the treatment we used a PIP scanner (Polycontrast Interference Photography) belonging to Harry Oldfield, a former science teacher who now devotes his time to researching healing. A PIP scanner is able to track in real time the movement of an energy field. Thus we were able to witness first-hand a visual energy record of a treatment given by Seka.

At the start of the treatment there was a heavy black energy cloud around the injured site, but during the healing it changed to a clear blue-and-green energy. Immediately after the session we also saw a discharge of very dark red energy from the centre of Seka's chest – around her heart. From what I know of how the human body regenerates and also from what I understand of human energy fields, I can surmise that Seka works by channelling a highly organized energy pattern, which allows tissues to return back to their original blueprint, their natural healthy state. I had just this one very powerful treatment with Seka, and after weeks of total loss of function, my wrist was fully functional within three days.

The fact that any human has this capacity to work so flexibly and so deeply with energy is testament to the possibilities for all of us who struggle with our limited experiences of the energetic world.

Dr Anthony Soyer, MB, BSc.

History and research show that the Western world has been investigating energy for longer than most people realize, but it's still not conclusive enough to persuade most scientists to invest their time and money in finding out how this subtle force affects health. But this is slowly changing. Whatever the label, it seems that there is definitely an energetic network that links the organs and systems of the human body. The great news is that some scientists have managed to research some practitioners like me who can affect the human energy field directly with their own power.

Bio-Energy Put to the Test

In the West the bulk of research into healing has been done in North America. In the 1960s at the McGill University School of Medicine in Montreal, Dr Bernard Grad, Associate Professor of Gerontology, conducted a series of in-depth experiments into the laying-on-of-hands. Healing goes by many names and under various guises, and these labels help to differentiate between the different types of work – for example, spiritual healing, crystal healing and psychic healing. I choose to use the term Bio-Energy because I feel that this term clarifies the scientific foundation of my practice, which isn't aligned to any religion or spiritual school. The laying-on-of-hands is in fact very similar in nature to my work.

Dr Grad used a Hungarian healer, Oscar Estebany, for his tests.[11] Estebany claimed that he had great success in dealing with thyroid problems so it was decided that he would start by treating thyroid goitres in mice. To make the mice ill, Grad put them on a low-iodine diet and also fed them an agent that is known to block thyroid function. Once their thyroids were enlarged, the mice were divided into four groups. One group received no treatment at all; another group was held by non-healers who attempted to heal; the third control group was wrapped in electrothermal tape to simulate the heat of human hands; and finally there was the treatment group. None of the treated mice were to have direct contact with Estebany's hands – instead, he held their container. After the experiment all of the mice showed an increase in thyroid size due

11 Richard Gerber, MD, *Vibrational Medicine: New Choices for Healing Ourselves* (New York 1988).

to the induced illness, but the Estebany group had a significantly slower rate of goitre development.

Grad used the same set-up to see if Estebany could heal wounds, and after cutting the mice's skin with wounds of the same size and depth, those treated by Estebany were left with either a tiny scar or none at all, whereas the control groups showed obvious scarring. The results of this experiment were published in the *International Journal of Parapsychology* and in the *Journal for the American Society of Psychical Research*, and Grad's work inspired others to investigate the mystery of healing.

Dr Justa Smith, a nun and biochemist based in New York, wanted to find out if healers could accelerate the rate of natural enzyme activity. She thought that if she could prove this, she would have found the most likely explanation for increased growth and healing. Dr Smith also used Estebany as her subject. She tested his effect on the digestive enzyme trypsin because it is relatively easy to track and measure any changes. Estebany held a test tube of the solution, and Smith took samples periodically as he worked. She tested the enzyme's ability to bring about a chemical reaction and found that Estebany was able to increase the enzyme rate, and that the longer he worked, the more rapid the rate became. Armed with these positive results, Dr Smith went on to test a number of different enzymes in the same way. She discovered that the rate of enzyme activity didn't always increase, and at first she was confused as to why Estebany's healing would slow the enzyme. What she soon realized was that the direction of change in the rate of enzyme activity when the healer worked was always in the direction that induced greater health in the body: he wasn't told what the enzymes were, so had no conscious idea of which direction to induce change – it was a natural healing instinct.[12]

I can relate to this sense of instinct. Over the years I have gained

12 Richard Gerber, MD.

a lot of medical knowledge, and I use it with the information I sense through my hands. But I wasn't always this knowledgeable. When I first started to heal, I worked purely on instinct and just trusted myself to bring about the best results possible.

We can see from these examples that there have been several scientific experiments that go some way to show the power of energetic therapies. I encourage my patients, where possible, to get medical tests done before and after their treatment. This isn't for my benefit – I know what I've done – but it helps some patients to cope with the psychological aspect of recovery.

One of my patients, Julia Campbell Carter, was suffering with Graves' disease, a thyroid condition. Julia had been very sceptical about my work. She had seen specialists in Germany and London. She had been prescribed drugs to inhibit the production of thyroid hormones and had taken these for fourteen months. She was also advised to take a further course of radioactive iodine drugs to destroy her thyroid, meaning that she would have to take artificial thyroid hormones for the rest of her life. That was when she decided that she had nothing to lose in coming to see me. She told *The Times*, 'I'm a lawyer, I'm a doubter, and I didn't believe in alternative medicine. But I was absolutely desperate.'

Julia was suffering from heart palpitations, cold sweats, stomachache, diarrhoea and she had lost nearly two stone in weight. She told the newspaper, 'I had a pulse of 140 beats per minute, which made me feel as if I had drunk several cups of very strong coffee. One terrible night I actually thought I was having a heart attack. I looked like a haggard old lady and felt dreadful.' She was in a pretty bad way.

I treated Julia for a week. I told her to take things as easy as she could, so that her body could get as much benefit from the treatments as possible. I knew that she would be OK after a month, but I always have to make sure I instil that faith in my patients. Julia told *The Times*, 'Seka said that in a month's time my blood results would be fine and I would no longer need to take the hormones. She was right. When I had a scan at the hospital a month later, it showed that my thyroid had nearly halved in size and my blood results were almost normal. After two more sessions all my symptoms, such as the heart palpitations and the digestive problems, had gone. I soon returned to my normal weight, and I've had no thyroid problems since.'

I have learned through my years of experience when a condition will heal, but as in Julia's case, it's good for the patients, and their doctors, to get proof of what Bio-Energy can do. For some people, the amazing experience of becoming free of negative symptoms and feeling so much better, sometimes after years of suffering, is a mental and physical challenge. People get used to being ill, so if the cure seems relatively sudden, it can be overwhelming.

Different Kinds of Healing

There are many healers who work in different ways from me. Some work with angels, or spirits guide them, and others work by directly channelling energy from a higher source. Because of the variety of healing methods, people can choose a type that they feel comfortable with, and the most important thing is that someone feels at ease and confident with the ability of the healer.

I have found that most new patients tend to have little hope that I can help them, and I don't mind people being cynical. I think it's healthy to question, and sceptics are often overjoyed with their results because they have such low expectations! Because I believe that there is a scientific element to Bio-Energy healing, I tend to attract patients who are sceptical about alternative therapies. Luckily, I don't need people to believe in what I do for it to work. The best examples I have of patients who have no belief or preconception of my work are children.

Children and babies are simple to treat because they don't have any other issues to get in the way of their treatment. I have treated several youngsters with asthma, and more recently I've seen an increase in the number of brain tumour cases. With these and other illnesses, adults can be distracted by stress and other mental barriers, and I often have to deal with lots of other problems before I can get to work on the main illness. With children, however, I can work directly with the condition.

I remember one case of a child who had advanced rheumatoid arthritis. It's very unusual to see a child with this disease, and it was one of the worst cases I've seen. The young boy had such swollen joints that he couldn't walk at all and was on heavy doses of steroids. All he knew was that he couldn't walk and that he was in a lot of pain, but he had no other understanding of what was going on. The treatments worked very well on him and he was able to walk unaided and come off his medication after five sessions. He was just so happy not to have any more pain and to be able to play like other children, and he didn't try to rationalize what had happened. It was so refreshing! In comparison, when I have worked with adults who have similarly severe cases of rheumatoid arthritis, it has taken several blocks of treatment over a number of months to achieve total recovery because as well as work on the arthritis, I have had to help them clear their fear, their stresses and their disbelief that they can be cured.

I have also worked with several epileptic children. One baby was brought by her parents from Croatia. She was only eight months old, and she had been born during the war. At three months old she had started to get fits, and her growth had been stunted by having fits every few minutes. The lack of oxygen to her brain meant that she couldn't develop at all. She had little chance of leading a normal life. We saw her change right from the first session. When her parents laid her on my treatment table, she was still and peaceful, and the treatment worked much more quickly than it would have done on an adult.

Hyperactivity is another common illness that I treat in children. I remember a pair of toddler twins who were brought in by their parents. The mother and father were shattered! The minute I saw them I noticed their weariness, and they looked relieved and amazed when each child in turn lay still and quiet as I worked on them. They were cured within the first couple of treatments because all I had to do was correct their energetic frequency. They had no mental barriers to remove, and they didn't question what I was doing. If only all cases were are simple as that.

One area where I have less experience but which also proves the same point is the treatment of animals. Whilst they are intelligent in their own way, most people will accept that animals don't have beliefs and make judgements in the same way that humans do. Animals are intuitive creatures: they can sense danger and fear and, equally, they have a capacity to sense when someone is friendly and harmless. And so the treatment of animals is an area in which it is easy to disprove the potential placebo effect of Bio-Energy healing. Like children, they relax and enjoy the comfortable feeling of the treatment. They seem to automatically trust me and that makes my life a lot easier.

Another area in which it's hard to argue the placebo effect is the treatment of sports injuries. As with Prince Andrew's ankle, when I have worked with sportsmen and women who have come with straightforward broken bones or muscle strains, the results are very clear to see. Injuries aren't psychosomatic – they're very tangible and it's these successes that have helped me to build long-term relationships with tennis players, footballers and athletes.

Levels of Healing

One fascinating thing I learned at the Institute of Bio-Energy Research is that as well as there being different kinds of healing there are also different levels of healing ability. The fact that there were enough other people with Bio-Energy powers to warrant formal categories of power meant that I wasn't a freak phenomenon! The reason I'm including this information is because I feel it's critical to the well-being of other practitioners to gain an understanding of their ability and of their limitations.

The institute had recorded four levels of healing. They took into consideration the practitioner's ability to transform energy, their degree of consistency and their level of resistance, all of which makes a lot of sense.

Levels of Bio-Energy Healing Power

Level of Power	Conditions that can be Treated	Reliability of Power
1	Headaches, muscular aches, etc.	Inconsistent and variable
2	Inflammation, early-stage rheumatism, etc.	Inconsistent and variable
3	Broken bones, later-stage rheumatism, etc.	Mainly constant
4	All illnesses: except AIDS, late cancer or some tumours, etc.	Constant

They found that not only was my power constant, but I also had an usually high resistance to electricity, so they created another level, level five, to rate, my gift. After running tests on me, the scientists discovered that I was often able to totally rid people of disease. I suppose I must have sensed I had a strong ability because I had already been working on extreme cases with excellent results.

My energy was consistent and constant, which meant that I supposedly didn't have any limitations on what I could work on.

The constancy of energy is a really important factor for healers. With healers who have an inconsistent gift, their energy switches on and off and this is out of their control. This means that if they're unaware that their power is 'off' when they're working, they may drain their patient and also cause themselves to be ill. In doing their best to help others, healers must be careful to look after themselves as well because their health is critical to their job.

Find Your Own Level

When we work at our optimal level, we find that we are happy, balanced and successful, but if we push ourselves too hard, we can often damage our energy. Let's take singing as an example. Everyone can sing. I'm a mediocre singer and I could be trained to sing better, but even with the best training in the world, I don't have what it takes to be a world-class opera singer. I just don't have a natural gift and if I pushed myself too hard, I'd probably damage my voice and everyone else's eardrums! The same applies to healing: everyone has healing ability. When a mother hugs her child, she is using her healing energy to comfort them but she's probably not aware of it. There are many people who have a stronger gift and they can reduce headaches or stomachaches – and I'd encourage them to use this power – but if they try to heal a more serious illness, they could damage their energy.

Another way to explain this is to draw parallels with things that are more familiar to us. If you replace a sixty-watt light bulb with a forty-watt bulb, it will be too weak to give adequate light, and if you use a hundred-watt bulb instead, you risk blowing the fuse. You have to find the right level of power for what you need. If you want to bake a cake and the recipe says that the oven should be

180°C, then by setting the temperature at 250°C you will burn it, and if you turn it down to 100°C, it won't cook. It has to be just right, and it's the same with healing energy. Energy has to be adjustable; and I automatically transform different frequencies according to what my patient needs. I can transform energies of very high and very low frequency, but this skill isn't easy to learn; I do it intuitively.

We all have things that we naturally do well, and when we work with these talents, everyone benefits. Everyone has different strengths, and when we each find our niche, we fit together perfectly, like a jigsaw. No particular talent or job stands out as any more important than another – they're all just different.

During my time in the UK I've seen an increase in the number of people who teach healing. I think it's great that there are schools to teach people how to be aware of energy – how to sense it, move it and to work with it – and if you're born with the ability to heal, then you can nurture this to its full potential. A practitioner's energy has to be spot on to be able to heal safely, so it's vital to be aware of this and to keep an eye on the effect that healing has on you.

I am lucky that I don't get drained any more from healing, but I can still become ill if I allow myself to get run down, and I need to be careful of this. It's better to err on the side of caution, and as much as I would like to be able to help everyone, there are times when it simply isn't wise for me to treat people. Sometimes Bio-Energy would be ineffective, and sometimes the potential risks of the treatment outweigh the benefits. It's hard to say no to someone, but their safety has to come first.

When to be Careful

The scientists in Milan told me to avoid treating anyone who has a pacemaker. Blood flow increases during the healing process, and

I'm comfortable with how this affects a natural heart. Some people claim that it's perfectly safe for pacemakers to take this pressure, but I'm not prepared to take any risks at all. For similar reasons, I also avoid treating anyone with varicose veins or thromboses. A vein differs from other tissue, such as muscle, because once it's damaged there is little that can be done to regenerate it. I am able to move clots, but that's not always easy and even destroying clots can be risky – and it's a chance that I won't take.

I also avoid treating women who are menstruating. When I first started working, I did treat women at all stages of their menstrual cycle, but over time I discovered that the body isn't able to absorb as much energy as usual at this time, which makes the treatments less effective. This can be a waste of time for my patient and for me, and sometimes the menstrual flow can become unusually heavy. This is the only time that Bio-Energy affects a function in the body other than the condition that's being treated, and whilst it's not dangerous, it's unnecessarily uncomfortable. A woman's body is naturally detoxifying itself during menstruation and so I feel that it's best to leave the body to do this without interfering. I also used to avoid giving treatments whilst I was menstruating, as I'd find myself getting drained, but I have learned to control this and am able to carry on working to my usual standard throughout my cycle.

I'm careful when it comes to pregnant women, although there is no particular danger in treating an expectant mother. There is so much mystery over what causes birth abnormalities, premature births and miscarriage that if anything were to happen to either mother or baby, it would potentially be easy to point the finger at alternative treatments. I would never want to be in a position where my work was implicated as the cause of any complication, so I feel that it's just safer to stick with what I feel comfortable and confident. I feel that I'm honoured to have such a gift and that I should only use it when I know it can definitely do good.

Healing Is Natural

Our bodies are healing all the time. When people don't believe that healing is possible, I want to tell them to think of a time when they cut themselves and saw how the body repaired itself in a matter of days. Healing is a natural phenomenon. Our bodies are continually renewing: we have new skin every month, a new stomach lining every four days and a new liver every six weeks. Whenever I think about this it seems clear to me that our bodies are designed to regenerate. We are continually dying and being reborn, and what I can do is speed up this natural process. We have to remember that we are made of Bio-Energy, so it's only natural to treat ourselves by balancing this energy. But despite the fact that we are designed to heal, Bio-Energy still provokes very mixed reactions. Some people are firm believers, some are adamant disbelievers, and others have no idea what to believe!

Healing and the Medical Profession

Medicine is one of the most respected professions: there are millions of medical professionals worldwide who dedicate their lives to caring for the sick and thousands of medical researchers who are continually searching for new or improved ways to treat and cure disease. Most of us have grown up with a strong belief in modern medicine and what it can achieve. We were most likely born in a clinical environment, and as we grew up and fell victim to bugs and sniffles, we were bundled off to our family doctor for a dose of antibiotics and some painkillers. Men in white coats with stethoscopes and nasty-tasting medicine: that's whom and what we have relied upon to get us this far in life.

In conventional medicine the human body is believed to be a

physical structure – a biochemical matrix made up of bones, organs, nerves, blood and other fluids, and connective tissue. The body is seen as a mechanical instrument, and changes in its physiology are seen as dependent solely upon the body's structure, which most believe to be predictable and orderly. By staying within these parameters, conventional, or allopathic, medicine can be said to be truly objective: conditions can be measured, tested and seen under a microscope. Medicine is a logical science, and in the West we are brought up to respect it and respond to it.

A lot of people think of conventional medicine as a definitive concept, rarely daring to question it. Most of us blindly put our faith in doctors, not knowing where else we would turn if it were to fail us. We don't have the knowledge to question what we're prescribed, and the years of study that it would take for us to learn about it ensure that the profession stays inaccessible and mysterious.

Science or Art?

Medicine is classified as a science because it can only be practised after years of intense study, but I believe that there is another dimension to medicine. Knowledge is subjective, but I believe that how it is applied is an art.

I used to find it hard to understand why doctors were often so narrow in their approach. It seemed to me that they look for symptoms and then cure them with medication. It would make me cross because I didn't know what I know now. Doctors in the National Health Service are in a catch-22 situation: they want to help – that's why they spent years studying hard – but they also need to meet their targets. GPs, in particular, are given such a short amount of time to see each patient that they literally cannot afford to invest time to look at the bigger picture. They have so many people to see and so much paperwork to deal with that they are left with a relatively small proportion of time to do their real job.

I am also told by many doctors with whom I work that there is a need for doctors to protect their reputation. As we become more and more litigious, like the Americans, there is a growing risk that by giving patients anything other than a worst-case scenario, doctors put themselves at risk of being sued. If they tell someone they'll regain full health and that isn't the case, they could find themselves in an unpleasant situation. Many people who are sick take their doctor's word as gospel. and I really do believe that by protecting themselves with their diagnosis, some doctors limit their patients' chances of recovery by setting their beliefs too low. Sad though it is, I think it's true. It takes a brave doctor who uses both their artistic and scientific skills to be able to give an holistic treatment.

When I went to see Seka for the first time, I had been suffering from an overactive thyroid for years. My symptoms were weight gain, fatigue, a fuzzy mind, hair loss, dry skin and, of course, a swollen thyroid gland. Rather unusually, my symptoms were more fitting to those of an underactive thyroid, but I had refused all medical treatment because it was making my symptoms worse. At one point my doctor even wanted me to have my thyroid removed, saying that if I didn't, I would need to take medication for the rest of my life. I refused both options and now I'm so glad I did.

I had got my condition to a sufficiently controlled point that I could be signed off treatment, but my doctor was unhappy that I was wasting his time. I then tried a number of alternative treatments, including reflexology, herbal remedies and kinesiology, which brought some improvement, but I was nowhere near feeling healthy. I had reached a point where I could live with my condition, but life was far from perfect.

I heard about Seka through several friends who had been to see her, all of whom had remarkable stories to tell. I thought I might as well give it a go.

Seka didn't know anything about my medical history or ailments. She didn't ask me any questions and started the treatment by putting her hands on my head. After about five minutes she promptly announced, 'Your thyroid is out of balance.' She was spot on.

During the session I felt deeply relaxed. I was surprised that Seka touched me very firmly as most hands-on healers don't touch you at all. Every few minutes Seka made a series of pulling motions around my throat, which made a clicking noise from her hand. She then went to my abdomen and told me I'd had a terrible trauma in that area, which had nearly killed me. This was true, many years ago I had had an emergency operation on my abdomen because my appendix had burst. I was told by the doctors that I nearly died and it took me months to recover from it. I still have no idea how Seka picked this up.

Seka then told me that I needed one more session to complete the work on my thyroid. During the second session, again, I felt deeply relaxed and Seka was making the same pulling motions and clicking noise with her hand. After the treatment I felt really spaced out for a couple of hours but totally at peace.

I was astonished to find that, after just two treatments, my thyroid gland was no longer swollen – it had been swollen my whole life! Even now, a year after seeing Seka, I still regularly put my hand to my throat and I can't believe it's flat!

I can't show any medical evidence of Seka's work because I had stopped my hospital sessions a long time before seeing her, but given that my doctor had suggested surgery or a radioactive drink to kill the thyroid cells, that goes some way to prove how much I had been suffering. Because of seeing Seka, I didn't need any medication or medical intervention.

Here's a funny thing: a little while ago I bumped into my old thyroid specialist. The last time I had seen him he had told me that I would end up in hospital very ill if I didn't continue to take thyroid medication. When I saw him, he recognized me straight away – and I could see the amazement on his face that I was clearly healthy and at a normal weight!

Since seeing Seka, my weight has stabilized, my hair has grown thicker, my skin is no longer dry, and I am full of energy. Now my thyroid is healthy and strong, and I feel really well.

Anne Jirschitzka

My Approach

The process of healing can take time, and the body can sometimes have a strong reaction to the energy – something known as the 'healing crisis'. As negative energy releases, some patients may feel the resistance of the energy as a painful pulling sensation, so I do like to warn people that this can happen. It's normal and it's actually a positive sign that blocks are releasing, but I've had people wonder if I'm making them worse! Some patients also feel sick when I treat them, and others can feel tired, but again, these are all normal, positive signs. ME is a good example as it's not unusual for patients to feel worse during the first three days, but they always feel better afterwards. There are rare occasions when I won't warn someone of what they might feel because I know that they'll be afraid and their fear can make the pain worse, but most times I'll give some indication.

I always tell my patients, 'I will do my best.' They don't need me to spell out to them exactly what will happen, they just need to have hope. Even when I sense that I can help someone to full recovery, I rarely tell them. They need to see it and feel it themselves, and when positive changes happen quickly, I feel a shift in their frequency to a level of more optimism and hope. Referred patients are the easiest to deal with because they tend to have a good idea of what I do and so they don't turn up afraid or overly sceptical.

If someone has been ill for a long time, I need to help them to build their beliefs so that they can accept the possibility of recovery. I remind them of how their body used to be, and this helps to reset the mind to a healthy point so that it can catch up with the changes in the body. For example, if someone has not been getting enough oxygen around their body, they've probably forgotten how it feels to have strong circulation and well-fed muscles, so the brain has to be reminded. I know it sounds strange, but when someone has been unwell for months or years, they have usually become so used to feeling and believing a certain way that it takes some consistent work to show them that their situation and body have changed. If this mindset doesn't shift, people risk dragging themselves back into their illness, and I will always distract my patients from any negative thoughts. Someone may say to me, 'Seka, what if I collapse?' because they're so used to this happening. To me, it's a ridiculous thought: they used to be able to walk or run and they probably never thought about collapsing then, so why should they think about that now?

How Good Can It Get?

Another difference I have noticed between allopathic medicine and many forms of alternative medicine is the end goal – the way that people want to feel when treatment is over. Most medical doctors will try to help their patients reach a point where they are free of negative symptoms – a neutral point. That may be acceptable for a lot of people, but who's to say that a neutral state is as good as it gets? In my mind, it doesn't automatically make sense that someone who has 'no symptoms' of heart disease is in the best health they can be, or that a state of 'no symptoms' of a stomach ulcer is conclusive evidence that a stomach is truly healthy and working at its optimum level. Think of it another way: just because we're not in debt doesn't mean we're rich, and by being rich, we're not automatically happy. The absence of one situation doesn't necessarily mean that another exists; therefore no sign of disease doesn't equal wonderful health. Whenever I treat someone, I aim to make them as rich in good health as I possibly can.

I always set myself a high benchmark. How do you know whether you feel the best that you can? If you haven't felt fantastic for years, it's hard to remember what it feels like. You may not have any negative symptoms, but that doesn't mean that you can't acquire positive ones. Does it make sense that just because there's no textbook or journal that describes a condition that it can't exist? We know that's not true.

We don't usually wait for our house to fall down before we decorate or for our car to stop working before we service it. If we waited for everything in life to fall into total disrepair or meltdown, then we would regularly experience periods of malfunction and standstill – which, funnily enough, is what many of us experience with our health. We don't pay attention to our fluctuations in energy, and we only sit up and take notice when our energy has run out, or our body has given up. By striving for the best state of health possible, we can avoid periods of breakdown.

To be in the best state of health, we have to address what's going on at all levels. The body's tissues are fed by oxygen, nutrients and a cocktail of chemicals, but they are also nourished by the energies and emotions within and around us. We have to look not only at the physical symptoms but also at our thoughts and feelings, and in my experience, most illness grows out of stress. By paying attention to our emotions and our stress levels, we may find the key to energy imbalances and, therefore, sickness. This is what I see as holistic healthcare.

Medicine is essential to our well-being and helps to alleviate and cure many symptoms of illness. But as many doctors will admit, modern medicine is a relatively young practice and it has its limitations. In the main, it neglects to acknowledge the existence of a vital force that animates the human machinery. Complementary healthcare practices maintain that the body has a spiritual domain as well as a physical one. It's without doubt that our bodily systems can and do malfunction, but mechanical faults occur because of changes at an energetic level – and these energetic shifts lead to the body's breakdown.

The two bodily realms are interconnected: our physical framework is nourished by our energy system, and I believe that the key to treating illness lies in the re-patterning and re-energizing of the energy field, which then affects the cells and functioning of the body. By dealing with emotional and mental components, alternative medicine is deemed to be subjective. It's hard to detect the existence of a higher level of matter, and it cannot be anatomically dissected, transplanted or monitored. But think about love: we can't see or touch it, yet we know it exists; we can't measure sadness, but we've all felt it at some time. Like these emotions, we can't see energy, but we know it's around us.

Illness has existed since the beginning of time. Although diseases have evolved and causes of illness may have changed, the human body has always been vulnerable to sickness. But it is only relatively recently that we have had a deep understanding of how the body works. Until then, healthcare professionals relied on intuition, and that intuition led to the first investigations into human energy. Not so many generations ago our ancestors relied on nature to heal them. They used herbs, roots and flowers as their medicines, and their practitioners were shamans and other healing figures. But whilst these origins are no longer the norm, they are still apparent, and many people nowadays are open to the power of alternative treatments.

Over the fifteen years that I've known Seka she has treated me for several ailments. One particularly memorable occasion was on a Sunday evening when I was cooking spaghetti. I went to lift the pot off the heat and the tea towel I was using caught on the stove, sending the entire pan of boiling water over my right hand and arm and leaving me very badly burnt up to the elbow. I screamed out in pain and my knees buckled under me from the agony and the shock. Luckily I still had the presence of mind to call Seka.

As was so often the case, Seka came to my rescue and gave me healing for over an hour. As she drew the excruciating pain out of my arm, the energy seemed to shift from my arm into her right hand. As she drew out my pain, her right hand turned a very dark shade of red, and when she flicked her hand, there was a clicking noise and the pain literally went away. After the healing, I was exhausted but elated that the pain was no longer intolerable. Seka and I were even able to enjoy a cold shot of vodka, which my husband poured us to get over the shock.

The next day I went to the burns unit at Chelsea and Westminster Hospital. Only one big blister had developed, which they cut open and treated accordingly. Seka continued giving me healing over a couple of days, and I was completely pain free after the second session. When I went for my last appointment at the hospital, they couldn't believe how quickly the new skin had formed and how well my arm had healed. I told them that I had had healing, but it didn't seem to register: either they didn't understand what I meant or they just didn't take it on board, but they did say, 'Whatever you're doing, keep doing it!' Apart from a faint white mark on the inside of my arm you would never know that I had been so badly burnt.

M.P.O.

How Do I Diagnose?

One of the areas in which I have managed to gain respect from doctors is my diagnostic ability. The thing that can make diagnosis tricky is the fact that there are often numerous causes for symptoms. When doctors take a medical history and examine a patient, they have many things to take into consideration and they may also use further testing. They often rely on what the patient tells them about their health and lifestyle, so the more they know, the more accurately they can diagnose. This whole process can take a fair amount of time, but it's critical in order to treat someone properly. For me, it's different. I can't explain why this works, but I can diagnose all energy blockages quickly and very accurately.

My hand acts as a scanner, and I simply run it down my patient's body a few inches away from them and wait to see what information comes to me. It's important that I empty my mind and become very relaxed. I never allow what I already know or what I initially see to affect my judgement, because I've learned over the years that the most accurate knowledge comes to me through my palms. I don't analyse or question; I just gather the facts.

When I first started to work, I didn't know what the various sensations in my hands meant, but after several years of treating people some very clear patterns started to emerge. For example, sometimes it can feel as if a knife is stabbing my hand, or it can feel like several knives are cutting me. As the pain gets stronger, my right hand, which draws out the negative energy, starts to change colour and becomes a purple-blue tone, a bit like a bruise. My left hand, which feeds in energy, doesn't change at all. When I shake my right hand, the pain reduces and it looks normal again. My hands can also ache or sting, and each feeling means something different, so as I became more experienced, I could tell what each kind of pain was telling me. It's like connecting to the Internet and receiving automatic downloads: once I connect to my patient, the information comes through.

I receive information about their physical state – where they have blocks of energy, inflammation, scars from old wounds or surgery – and I also gather facts about their life, including things that have happened to them in the past that are now affecting their health. It's as if I'm reading a poem of their life – I see pictures and get messages and I only receive information that I need. For some reason, I only get what's necessary.

Often I find energy blocks that have been caused by suppressed emotional memories, and I usually warn my patients that this may happen so they don't get a surprise. These emotional blockages are like closed doors: while they remain shut, I can't heal the illness. People are often afraid to face these events again, so I talk them through the pain and help them to recognize it. Once they have recognized and faced these old memories, they are able to open the door to healing and I can work on them.

What I also learn from the diagnostic scan is what needs treating in the body most urgently. Sometimes people have one root problem and many symptoms. This is often the case with ME sufferers. They are experiencing a huge list of complaints, such as headaches and candida, but I know that by working on the neurological malfunction, their whole body will benefit and the symptoms will disappear. This may mean telling a patient about a condition of which they were unaware, but it's important to do so in order for them to experience optimum health. For example, someone may come to me because they're suffering from headaches, but I can tell that they have rheumatoid arthritis, which is much more of a priority. In cases like these I have to tell someone what's going on in their body so that they understand what I'll work on: it's hard for me to treat a minor ailment when something more serious needs my attention.

I had a client the other day who didn't want to tell me about himself. He knew exactly what was wrong with him, but he wouldn't tell me anything. He wanted to test me because he was very cynical about my gift. I wanted to win his trust so that he'd be confident in my ability, so when I scanned him, I brought up every single thing I found, and he was astounded. There was a great deal going on in his body – and luckily, he was aware of all the problems – and it proved to him that I can diagnose well.

I have been treating a blind man for some time now. He told me that he had been diagnosed eight years ago with hysterical blindness, a psychosomatic, stress-related condition. I knew straight away that this wasn't right. He actually had a blockage in the back of the brain that had genuinely affected his vision. Since he started his treatments he has had another opinion, which turned out to be the same diagnosis that I had given. It took a while for the shock to sink in, as he was so upset that he had been receiving the wrong treatment for eight years, but I helped him to see the positive in the situation: what else was there to do? He couldn't turn back the clock so we talked about how he had developed his other senses over that time and how his situation had led him to do lots of charity work. Since I started working with him his sight has improved by about 50 per cent and he no longer needs to carry a white stick. With such good results, it was time for him to move on, not to apportion blame or be bitter. Even though he had told me what his diagnosis had been, I have learned to trust my own information – because it's usually right.

Unless I absolutely have to, I avoid telling my patients about the specifics of any of their problems. I just talk about blockages and focus my attention on clearing their energy. But you wouldn't believe how many people are disappointed by this! They want me to give them a long list of ailments and to label every single symptom they have. So many people want to justify the way they feel, and a few even enjoy being victims of an illness. I have learned not to make this any worse by sharing what I see: more often than not, I can work without communicating the negative.

The Results Speak for Themselves

One of my great friends and long-standing patients is Paul McKenna, the world-renowned hypnotist, who has kindly written the foreword to this book. Paul is incredibly open about trying alternative health practices and is more aware than most people of how powerful the mind can be. However, although Paul supports and believes in my work, a few years ago his father wasn't quite as confident in my abilities as he is now!

I had been suffering from a heavy cold and chest infection, both of which had left me weak. During the three months that followed this bad bout of illness the power in my legs, arms and hands got weaker. I was referred to a consultant for tests and was told I had rheumatoid arthritis and that my case was about as bad as it could get. Eventually I could hardly walk and didn't even have enough strength to open the car door. One night my wife got a broom for me to use as a crutch so I could climb the stairs to bed. I kept thinking that I'd soon be in a wheelchair.

My son Paul was insistent that I go and see a healer who he rated very highly. Having always been a man who believed in conventional medicine, I was somewhat sceptical: I couldn't see how this lady could help me. But Paul can be very persuasive and I ended up giving in to him. I agreed to meet Seka but I had low expectations.

At the first treatment Seka stood in front of me and slowly moved her hands over and around my body. My right arm suddenly started to shake uncontrollably, and I felt a rushing sensation down my arm to the fingertips, where the feeling seemed to disappear. Seka then asked me to lie down for the rest of the treatment. She explained that something had unblocked, but I had no idea what that 'something' was. She was convinced I'd soon be better, but I didn't realize quite how soon that would be!

That night I could walk freely and I felt strong. I didn't feel any pain at all. I kept saying to everyone, 'What has Seka done? How does she do this?' I was amazed and overjoyed. After two more treatments I felt so good I came home and mowed the lawn – an unthinkable activity considering how immobile I'd been for three months! After the fifth and final treatment I was completely back to normal.

Nobody is more convinced than me of Seka's healing power. I head straight to see her if I have a problem, and I visit her regularly just for energy top-ups. I always recommend Seka to anyone with a health issue, which is quite something given what a cynic I was. I've learned from my own experience that we should all take a more open view of the many alternative practices that are available. I decided to try something different and I now have a new perspective. I'm an advocate of Bio-Energy and would recommend everyone to try it.

Bill McKenna

Paul wrote about his father's recovery in his book, *The Paranormal World of Paul McKenna,* and it's interesting to see this case from his side: 'A few years ago my father began to suffer from rheumatoid arthritis. The Dean of Rheumatology who was treating him at a major London hospital had told my father that his blood tests showed him to be about as badly affected as it was possible to be [. . .] after he had seen Seka for a course of treatments, the effect was dramatic. "That healer worked!" he declared. "I feel fantastic." It was obvious. Indeed, he looked younger, and his energy and optimism had returned. I asked him what the Dean of Rheumatology had said, and he replied that although it defied explanation, the latest blood tests indicated that all traces of the illness had completely disappeared.'

Whilst Bill's doctor was willing to admit that he was unable to explain how the illness had been abated, it has become apparent to me during years of communication with doctors that in spite of clear positive results, some people still need explanations. Sometimes things just can't be explained in readily accessible ways, but that doesn't mean that their results don't speak for themselves.

I'm in the very fortunate and satisfying position of having hundreds of testimonials and letters from patients who have experienced recovery from illness and injury. It would seem logical that such positive results and successful case studies would help to convince the medical world of the power of Bio-Energy healing, however, we have yet to reach a stage whereby it is considered a mainstream practice.

I treated Linda Campbell, wife of radio presenter Nicky Campbell, after she was hit by a golf ball that shattered her sunglasses into her right eye. The glass was removed from her eye, which began to heal, but she was still in agony and started to experience other symptoms: pains in her neck and lower back, constant diarrhoea, a persistent fever, insomnia, swollen lymph glands, loss of appetite and paralysis in her right arm and leg. After tests by her GP it seemed that the injury to Linda's eye had been so bad that her brain had failed to function properly, and as a result, her immune system had stopped working. She had contracted a rare viral disorder that had led to ME.

As a last resort Linda made an appointment to see me and saw a vast improvement after one treatment. Linda's case was reported in *Today*. She told them, 'I cannot describe what happened to me except to say the effect was immediate and profound. For the first time in months I could walk unaided, and I slept properly that night for the first time in twelve weeks and could eat. It was a miracle . . . My own GP was astonished.'

Bio-Energy healing can help the overwhelming majority of patients, and by opening up their mind to their behaviour and emotions, the treatment also goes some way to preventing relapses and further illnesses. When we can succeed in opening up the minds of doctors and scientists, we will reach a much more integrated and holistic health service.

I have met Ms Nikolic and am impressed by her openness and professionalism. What she is doing seems to be quite remarkable, yet there is clearly no way in which we can measure what this is. What is interesting from my point of view is that with two exceptions all of the (fifteen to twenty) patients that I have referred to her have had clinical ME for periods as long as six or eight years and the improvements that they are experiencing at her hand have been not only in their energy levels but in the whole constellation of symptoms that characterize this puzzling condition . . . Unfortunately, the bigotry of a lot of our medical colleagues means that treatments which palpably have a beneficial effect are automatically rejected if the mechanism is not understood or appears in any way bizarre.

Dr David Lewis

A Happy Ending?

Conventional and complementary healthcare can work together to achieve the best results and to form a greater integrated concept of medicine. In Poland Bio-Energy healing has been an approved supplement to allopathic medicine since 1982.[13] While the medical profession in the UK is not as progressive as this, there are a steadily growing number of doctors here who can see that there are advantages to be gained from working in synergy. A significant proportion – about half – of my patients are referred to me by their doctor and one independent survey stated that 40 per cent of GPs

13 Milton Friedman, 'Mietek Wirkus Brings Bio-Energy Healing to America', *New Realities*, July/August 1987.

are happy to refer their patients to a complementary therapist, with some 20 per cent offering such therapies on their premises. It is also said that 75 per cent of NHS patients would like to use complementary therapies, so the situation is beginning to change but it may take time.[14]

14 Dr Michael Dixon, 'Best of Both Worlds', *Observer*, 22 July 2000.

4

THE INCURABLE AND THE UNIMAGINABLE

Over the years I've seen many people and treated many conditions. I've had patients who come to me just for a boost when they've got a lot going on, and at the other extreme I see people whose energy is so off balance that their body has given in to serious illness. I don't discriminate about whom I treat, but I do like to feel that my time is best spent treating people who find it hard to get relief through conventional medicine or those who wish to avoid invasive measures.

ME is a good example of an illness where I feel I can make a real difference. The medical profession has difficulty in treating some of the symptoms of the disease, and these are the symptoms with which I have most success: muzzy head, lack of concentration, exhaustion and collapses in energy.

I heard of Seka through an article in the *Guardian*. It couldn't have come at a better time as I was at my wits' end, having been getting weaker and more ill for nine years. I was mostly confined to bed, unable to walk, and, in addition, I was getting endless frequent migraines and my spine was becoming increasingly distorted and painful as a result of old injuries and my lack of muscles. No other treatment had helped and I had tried everything.

At the initial diagnostic session Seka assessed the energy field around my body. She said that I was very ill and had such problems that she was doubtful that she could do much for me, which was very honest. However, I was desperate and persistent, so she agreed to have a go.

Within the first few treatments my spine straightened up quite a bit. I was amazed. Since then I have had two more blocks of treatment and am going for my fourth block. The improvement, though slow, is sure. I am sleeping well for the first time in years. I have a little bit more energy; I am doing more and can now do tiny exercises to build up my non-existent muscles, so eventually my back will straighten out completely. A bicep was spotted recently. The migraines are less frequent and will diminish as I get stronger.

Although I am still in a pretty bad state and have a long way to go, compared to last year my condition is brilliant. Altogether I feel I am not doing too badly for a write-off.

G. H.

Infertility

Infertility is another example of an area where I like help because patients invest several months, even years, undergoing what can be very stressful and disturbing treatments, not to mention the financial cost.

I treated a lady called Sophie Gough just after she'd had an ectopic pregnancy. She had been receiving hormone treatment for several months to help her to ovulate and as a result of the ectopic pregnancy she had suffered from a ruptured fallopian tube. A leading IVF specialist told her that she had to have surgery or start IVF straight away if she wanted any chance of conceiving. Sophie wanted to avoid the stress of IVF at all costs and so she decided to try an alternative treatment and came to see me.

I knew as soon as I ran my hands over her body that she had a physical blockage in her remaining fallopian tube. I also knew she had a good chance of conceiving naturally once this was gone so I worked to clear the blockage. Sophie was pregnant within a month of having her first treatment but sadly miscarried after eleven weeks. Both Sophie and I knew that she was able to conceive naturally but that her energy needed more tuning to be at the strongest frequency possible for her to have a child. She continued to see me for booster treatments, and three months later she was pregnant with her son Louis.

Sometimes it is impossible for someone to conceive naturally, but what is often diagnosed as infertility is often suppressed fertility. In most of the cases that I have treated, medical tests have failed to show any biological reason why a man or woman can't conceive – and that's when it's important to look at the person's emotional health.

Stress and fear of not conceiving are major factors in suppressing fertility. These negative emotions send the wrong messages to your body: no matter how much you might want a baby and no matter how much time you spend thinking about it, your subconscious mind picks up on the energy of these negative emotions and reads them as a sign that you don't want to conceive. This is the case for men as much as it is for women, as stress can affect a man's sperm count. Once you become desperate to conceive, your body chemistry alters, making it very difficult for pregnancy to happen.

The key thing to do to conceive successfully is to focus on anything but conceiving. You have to distract yourself from what you're scared of, and once you stop putting pressure on yourself, conception is much more likely to happen. It's very common for couples who have successful IVF treatments to go on to conceive naturally: once they no longer put themselves under pressure to have a baby, their energy starts to vibrate at the correct healthy level. But whether it's stress-induced or whether it's for a biological reason, I have a great success rate in this area.

Cancer

Another condition that I can sometimes help when conventional routes can't is cancer. Cancer is a major killer across the world with one in three people suffering from some form of the disease during their life. Scientists have been looking for a miracle cure for many years and, although there are people who manage to defeat the illness using conventional medicine, there are still too many people dying because of this illness.

I used to avoid treating cancer patients because I was so in awe of this menacing disease. I knew how much people suffered, and in those days I wasn't confident that I could help them enough to make the treatments worthwhile. I lacked experience with cancer, and it took me a number of years to realize that I'd never gain this experience if I kept avoiding it. So I began to work with cancer sufferers. Over the years I have treated patients who are suffering at all stages of the disease.

If cancer is caught quickly, I can help restore someone to full health, but it is one of the few illnesses that is much more difficult for me to help them achieve total recovery in the very late stages. When the cancer is in these late stages, I can help someone enough for their blood tests to show improvement but only for as long as they come to see me. It means that they are as dependent on me as much as they are on their drugs, and this is a hard situation to deal with – both for them and for me.

Another challenge with cancer is that patients may be suffering from secondary cancer and can become susceptible to other illnesses as their immune system becomes weakened. I will instinctively focus on the area that needs the most urgent attention, as that's what my energy is drawn to. What's important is to help minimize pain where possible and also to relieve other symptoms. I never used to think that this was enough, but after working on a few cases I realized how much difference this makes to the patient and to those closest to them.

Seka had helped me recover from ME. The following year a close friend, who had seen my own remarkable recovery, arranged an appointment for his wife to see Seka. His wife's health had steadily declined over a period of six months, and despite her dreadful state and numerous medical tests and consultations, her doctors were unable to diagnose the problem.

When I saw the couple a few days after Seka's treatment, they both used the word 'miracle' as the only way to describe the effect. A woman who had been worn down to a very sad state after months of pain and exhaustion was now a picture of radiant health. She told us that she now felt just as she remembered feeling twenty years before at the age of thirty.

For about six weeks she had a wonderful life. But Seka's treatment had come too late to prevent the inevitable: her health started to decline again, and this time an advanced state of cancer was diagnosed, soon leading to her death. But as a close friend who saw them frequently until the end, I know that they both remained immensely grateful to Seka for giving six weeks of wonderful life to a woman who was already in a terminal condition.

Peter

When I first started to treat cancer patients, I had to face the fact that I may not have the success rate I'd had so far. Up until then I'd been able to help most patients completely overcome their illnesses so it was tough for me to contemplate a recovery rate of less than 100 per cent. Until this point I hadn't had to face the emotional trauma of being defeated and it took me a while to accept this possibility and to learn that I had to protect myself from the pain.

One particularly difficult case was with a seven-year-old boy who had been suffering with leukaemia since he was three years old. He was referred to me by a dowser, Alf Riggs, who had been called in by the child's parents to dowse their home, which was next door to a power station. The disease was very advanced, and I was treating the boy regularly. He showed such bravery during our sessions. He loved the way my jewellery jangled as I worked, and he would look forward to his treatment so he could entertain himself by playing with my bracelets and bangles. We built up quite a rapport and grew rather charmed by each other. Unfortunately, the cancer was too advanced to cure. Although doctors had given him a matter of weeks to live, I managed to prolong his life for a year and dramatically reduce his pain during that time. I found it hard to stay free of emotion watching this small child suffering in agony. His family invited me to the funeral, but although I had played a significant role in the last year of his life, I couldn't bring myself to go.

I believe, however, that miracles can happen and maybe one day I'll be able to heal a condition that I haven't yet healed. If I gave up because of my past experiences, I'd never find out and I could be denying someone a healthy recovery. I know this because although I avoided cancer for years because of my own fear, I have now helped heal a significant number of cancer sufferers.

Of all the cancers I treat, prostate cancer is one of the most common and also one of the easiest forms to treat. It tends to affect men who are in their late fifties to early sixties, and despite the high recovery rate, most men are very afraid of the disease. Some patients come to me after they've had chemotherapy, and others have Bio-Energy at the same time. Because chemotherapy is very draining on the body's energy reserves, I usually find that it's best to treat someone in between their chemotherapy sessions to help them recover, and with the combination of Bio-Energy and conventional medicine, almost all cases have a very successful outcome.

I could easily have carried on protecting myself from hurt and failure, but because I was prepared to give it a go, I have managed to give life to more people. And there's a chance that I still don't know what I'm fully capable of.

The Unusual . . .

There have also been a number of cases of people suffering with conditions that are as serious but much less common than cancer – diseases that you would never imagine existed.

In close-knit communities many patients are referred to me through their social networks rather than through their doctors, and after being in London for a few years, I had developed strong connections with many close ethnic groups. At the heart of one such group was an Indian family who ran a pharmacy close to my home in North London. They recommended me to friends of theirs, who travelled from India with their eighteen-month-old baby. I had been told that the child had been born not only with a hole in her heart but also without an outside layer of skin. She was in such a delicate condition that she had to travel in a glass cot, similar to an incubator. Before the family arrived I had no idea what to expect, but I knew the case was going to be a difficult one. As it turned out, I had no idea quite how harrowing it was going to be.

We hear horror stories of people being skinned alive and we can really only imagine what a person without skin looks like, but the reality was worse than anything I'd pictured: the baby's fingers were webbed, and her whole body looked raw, as if she'd been scalded in boiling water. I could see her tiny veins and bones through the finest layer of membrane. She looked so vulnerable that I didn't know where to focus, so as I treated her, I concentrated on her eyes. They were huge in comparison to the rest of her body, and they jumped out of her face and stared at me, pleading for help and relief from the agony.

I have never experienced anything quite like it. Over the week I watched as the baby's fingers started to separate and her skin began to form. The fresh new skin seemed to appear from nowhere, rather like when 'skin' forms on a hot milky drink as it cools down. By the end of the treatments she still looked delicate but much less vulnerable and raw. It had been truly remarkable to see such visual healing take place.

Another unusual and extreme case took place when I was in Sarajevo. I was still working in the marketing company and had yet to begin healing professionally, so I was relatively inexperienced. One day one of my colleagues called me in a terrible panic. A friend of his had had an industrial accident and acid had burnt her face. With burns, it's essential to start treating someone as soon as possible to avoid scarring. In this case, I was able to reach the lady in just over an hour. I visited her in hospital every day for seven days and, as with the baby, I watched the skin re-forming as I treated her. I still hadn't learned how to limit the pain I experienced, so I felt an intense burning and stinging in my face. Sadly, the accident had been so severe that she still completely lost one of her eyes, but I helped to save the other eye, and to the amazement of the doctors, her skin healed without a single scar. These cases are astounding, but others are just plain funny.

A seventy-nine-year-old man came to me because he was suffering from digestive problems. When he walked into my room, I was shocked by the size of his stomach. Even when he lay down for his treatment, the mass of his belly didn't seem to flatten out. As I worked on his abdominal area, the man's stomach started to cramp and lurch around and his eyes rolled back in his head. I was petrified that he was having a heart attack, so I asked him if he was OK. He said he was absolutely fine and so, not knowing what else to do, I carried on treating him. Afterwards my legs were shaking and I had to go out of the room for a glass of water. When I returned, I told my patient that I'd been worried about his reaction and that I thought the treatment might have been too much for him. Because he could see how afraid I was of having hurt him, he was completely honest with me and admitted that he'd actually been having an orgasm. I didn't know what to say – I was just so relieved that it wasn't a heart attack!

. . . and the Inexplicable

I've spent a great deal of time wondering whether to tell this story because, even now, I still find it hard to believe. But I think it's fascinating, and no matter what I write about, people will pick and choose what they believe. So I've decided to include all of the information in order to give a complete picture of my work – and I do have some reliable witnesses.

A scientist came to see me because of a persistent pain in his shoulder. As I began to treat him, my hands felt like they were in water – a feeling I have never had since. Usually, I feel a sensation of working my hands through honey or glue, but this time my hands seemed to move with more fluidity. This guy's reaction was also unlike anything else I had seen before or since. My patients usually feel very relaxed, and occasionally some people feel a bit of resistance as their energy starts to unblock, but on the whole the reactions are positive. This man writhed about on the bed. I could deal with that but what I found extraordinary was that his larynx leapt out of his throat like a frog, his bones made the most alarming cracking noises, and he was howling like a wolf. It was like a scene from a horror movie, and although it sounds almost funny now, at the time there was absolutely nothing amusing about the situation. Once I realized that it wasn't a joke, I nearly died from the shock.

I paused to ask him if he was OK, not wanting to draw too much attention to what was happening in case he was oblivious to it. He said everything was fine, and as he spoke, his body went back to its normal state, like a videotape on rewind. I've seen some amazing special effects in the movies, but I've never seen anything like it in real life. As soon as I started to treat him again, all the alarming symptoms started back up.

The staff at the clinic didn't know what to do. They knew not to disturb me during a treatment, and given that they could only hear what was going on, they presumed the man was just in a lot of pain. They couldn't see what I could see. I was in shock for hours afterwards and explained what had happened. We decided that on the following day my brother Momo, who is also a healer, would be in the treatment room with me and that a doctor, my good friend Dr Anthony Soyer, would be just outside. The same thing happened. Momo went pale and left the room, and Anthony said that he felt chilled to the bone due to the sound the man was making. We had agreed that they wouldn't interrupt me unless I called for them – and they're eternally grateful that I didn't! I was so afraid that still I didn't say anything to the patient for fear he would do something to me, so I continued to treat him for the rest of the week as normal. I have never been more relieved to see the back of someone.

To this day I can't explain what went on. His energy was unlike any human energy I've ever felt. I can only think that, being a scientist, he had an ability to alter his energy and that he was experimenting with me. I have had many scientists show an interest in my work, but it's always been for bona fide reasons and they've always approached me directly. I still get an eerie feeling when I think about this wolf man. I'm happy to say that this episode really was a one-off experience and, luckily, it happened to me when I had been healing professionally for a number of years. If it hadn't been for the witnesses that I'd called on and the staff at the clinic, I would have doubted my own sanity.

My Safety Mechanism

Many of my patients see me as a safe and comforting place when they are vulnerable and facing difficult times, but even when I bond with them, I have to remain as objective as possible. If I allow myself to become too emotionally involved, I find it hard to keep my energy strong and then I can't help them as best I can. When I first started healing, and before I understood how it could affect my energy, I would sometimes get attached to my patients. They would put their trust in me, and I thought that to do the best job, I had to open up to them. Then I learned that this was no good for either of us.

One of the most important things I've learned, and something that I also think is vital for our health, is that if we want to help someone, we have to stay emotionally detached from their illness or problem. When we're close to someone, we can't help but be emotionally involved with them: when they're ill, we suffer with them. If we allow ourselves to empathize, we lose our ability to think rationally and it's important that we see the positive side of the situation – not the worst-case scenario. By feeling their pain, we're no help to them at all, so we have to rise above the emotion to see what's really happening – that's how we can truly help. I can see up to twenty patients in a day, so I have to detach myself from them all, otherwise I'd be an emotional wreck!

We have to step back from the situation and observe it, as if we're watching from the outside. This helps us to be much closer to someone because when we're detached, we can make the best decision. One of the best examples of this is when parents take on their children's pain. The hardest person for me to treat is Bojan, my son. Suffering with your child is a natural part of being a parent, but it's not necessarily useful. We can only be strong when we stand apart from the emotion.

The more serious cases are very challenging for me and can be extremely rewarding. But when I treat someone who's in a lot of pain or discomfort, I realize more and more that prevention is a key component of healthcare. That's not to say that people who get cancer wouldn't get it if they'd lived differently, or that children wouldn't be born with unusual conditions – what it does say is that by being more aware of our energy and its changeability, we could become aware of disease at an earlier stage, when there's a higher chance of recovery.

5

NO LIMITS

When I first started healing, I didn't know anything about the optimal number of times to treat someone or how long I should treat them for. It didn't take me long to work out that not everyone would be healed after just one session, like Faroq was, so I just worked on people until they got better. When I was at the Scientific Institute for Bio-Energy Research in Milan, I learned that most people can only handle between twenty and thirty minutes of energy before their body becomes overloaded. Over time I worked out the structure that works best for my patients and for me, and for a while now I have been treating people in the same way: there is an initial block of five sessions on consecutive days and then many people return for booster treatments every few months. I found through trial and error that an initial intense period of healing works best. The patient is usually more focused and can put aside that one week to concentrate on their health, and the body responds well because each treatment builds on the previous one.

I've always had patients come to see me from all over the world, so if people are travelling from a long distance, it's easier for them to spend the week in London than make the trip on a weekly basis. This format suits many people, but for others, time or distance can be limiting factors. In cases where someone is too far away to come in person for a week of treatment, distance healing becomes an option.

I first discovered I could heal from a distance by accident. I was still in Sarajevo, so it was early on in my career. I was treating people at work, and my employers had given me a room to work in. One of my colleagues came into the room, and I motioned with my hand for him to lie on the couch. He jumped in shock and said, 'I felt that!' My energy was already channelling, and by directing him, he had felt the energy from my hand. I was a bit surprised, but by this time I was quite used to unusual things happening, so it didn't seem that ridiculous. I started experimenting by working on people with my hands just a few inches away from them. Then I tried from across the room. I moved to the next room, and then I was working on people on the other side of the city. It didn't take me long to work out that space wasn't an issue, and I built up the confidence to work on people from any distance.

How Distance Healing Works

Many people find the idea of healing hard to understand, but the concept of distance healing, also known as 'absent healing', can be even more difficult for them to come to terms with, so let me describe what I do as simply as possible.

When I'm doing a distance-healing session, I find a quiet place in which to sit and think about my patient. I find it easiest to explain to people if I use the analogy of making a telephone call: just as you need someone's telephone number to be able to connect with and call them, I need an image of someone so that I can connect to their energy. If I already know them, then I have their image in my head, but for people I haven't met before, I need to have their photo. They also need to be aware of when I'm treating them so they can connect back to me – rather like picking up a telephone receiver. If you telephone someone and they don't answer, there is no connection so you can't talk. It's the same with distance healing: if my patient doesn't connect to me, there's no line of communication.

It's best that both my patient and I are in a safe place, so I always recommend against driving during treatments. I usually ask people to sit or lie down, as a lot of people want to sleep after a distance-healing session, and it can be inconvenient or even embarrassing to be caught out in public!

One of my patients went to the cinema at the time when I said I'd treat her. She figured that she'd be sitting down somewhere safe so it should be OK. As the treatment started, she began to rock backwards and forwards in her seat and couldn't stop herself. She was mortified, and because she didn't want to move, she just sat there, rocking, for half an hour. It's also not unusual for patients to feel very warm and tingly or even for their limbs to levitate. You can see now why I suggest people find a quiet, safe place.

I sit and focus on that person and feel the same things as if I were treating someone in person. I use my hands as I would for a normal treatment and, unfortunately, I experience the same sensations and pains as usual, and my patients tend to feel very relaxed and at peace. This gives you some idea of what happens in practice, but to have a deeper grasp on how distance healing works in theory, we have to look back to science.

Human Waves

Electromagnetic waves travel at the speed of light, which means that they move from one place to another in a split second, no matter how far they have to go. Think about how many everyday things rely on a similar instant transmission of energy: we switch television channels from the other side of the room; we talk on the phone to friends who live hundreds of miles away and we watch live events from the other side of the world on television. Another example is the invisible communication we experience from person to person, which also involves energy moving across space. You may have experienced this when you've thought of someone, only for them to ring you a second later, or you might have been chatting to someone about a mutual friend, when they send you an email. These are all examples of how energy can communicate over distance.

Radio waves work in a similar way. Transistor radios used to be the most common wireless communications device, picking up signals from aerials at a great distance. Today the technology behind the basic radio is the foundation for almost every wireless device that we use: mobile phones, cordless phones, pagers, microwave ovens, televisions, GPS systems, wireless clocks, electric garage doors, baby monitors, wireless Internet networks and satellite communication. Energy doesn't know whether it's travelling a few metres or several hundred kilometres, and when we're on the receiving end, we take these things for granted and don't question the science behind them.

As I explained in Chapter 3, each one of us has our own particular frequency that radiates from us in the form of a wave, and these waves can be compared to radio or electromagnetic waves. Our energy waves are also unaffected by distance, and because my energy is consistently strong, I can tune into people's frequencies from great distances – and that's the basis of how this kind of healing works. I prefer to have physical contact with a patient to achieve the best connection, but it's not essential. Several patients of mine who have lit candles during their distance treatments have told me that the flame moves during the session – so people's reactions are as different as they would be when I'm treating them in person.

Dear Seka,

I am sorry that I took so long to write to thank you for giving me my life back. Since I saw you in March I have, for the most part, felt like a normal human being – something I hadn't experienced in five years. With the help of you sending energy on two occasions, I have maintained my good energy level. Although I can't play tennis due to this lingering 'tennis elbow', I do exercise in the swimming pool and ride my bike (again, for the first time in five years). I have also been able to take long walks when we go to the beach. The pressured feeling in my head is gone, and my memory is so much improved. I can also dial a telephone without mixing up the numbers! On those occasions that you sent me energy when I've felt low, I have improved and returned to feeling healthy.

I want you to know that I think of you very often and I thank you for my life, my health and my energy.

I have had some severe stresses in my life since March, and I have been able to make it through without relapsing. Prior to seeing you I would have been sick for weeks over any of the incidents. So again, thank you, thank you so very much. I sing your praises at every opportunity. I look forward to hearing from you.

Sincerely,

J. H.

PS This is the most I've written in five years.

Group Healing

Not only can I heal at a distance but I can also treat more than one person at a time. When I'm focusing on any group I either have to be in the room with them or I have to have their photos in front of me. The treatment works along the same lines as a conference call with everyone 'dialling in' at the same time: just as each person has to pick up the receiver to be a part of the call, my patients need to be conscious that I'm working on them, and again I always ask that they sit or lie in a quiet place and relax for the duration of the session.

One of my patients, Sandy, came to see me from South Africa. She stayed in London for the usual five-day block of treatment. When she got back to South Africa, many of Sandy's friends were interested in my work, so she asked me if I would do a distance healing session for a group. I agreed and Sandy helped me to organize it. Sandy collected a photograph from each person and arranged mutually convenient times on three consecutive days because five days was too hard to arrange. Each patient was to write a note to me after each session, telling me how he or she was feeling. A month after the sessions were over, Sandy did one last check on everyone and sent me a fax telling me how everyone was doing:

P. F.: Nausea gone. Many thanks for the healing!

P. C.: Remarkable improvement overall.

N. C.: Very well this week. Felt glowing after receiving energy. Grateful thanks to Seka!

D. S.: General improvement with ups and downs. But now working a full, busy day! (And clearing bush at plot in mountains on Saturday!)

M. N.: Generally better, although has had cold. Recovers from setbacks faster.

R. D. B.: Treatment wonderful, miraculous! Felt well enough yesterday to do washing by hand. So grateful to Seka for wonderful healing – after twenty-four years of suffering. (Sandy adds a note 'The joy and wonder in her voice were truly something to hear.')

E. F.: OK. Still off all tablets. Painted daughter's room at weekend. Lay down to receive healing on Thursday, then fell asleep thru it. But felt

marvellous the next day! Signs of starting to menstruate again naturally
– some spotting and cramps.'
Everyone has benefited so much, even those who don't seem to want
to admit it!
Thanks,
Sandy

My good friend Dr Anthony Soyer was part of a distance-healing
group that I ran over a month-long period. I was interested to
know how he'd found it, and he told me that it was clear when
the treatment started. He said, 'I felt like I was in a "love storm!"
I felt a cool energy and also a sheet of warmth – as if I was being
hugged. Then I felt tremendously energized.' That sounded good
to me.

The largest group of people I've worked on at once was during
a seminar called Extended Sensory Performance. I had been
invited to run this with Michael Breen, who is a trainer of neuro
linguistic programming, and Joe Moneagle, a remote viewer. There
were 300 delegates, and Michael had asked me to demonstrate my
healing powers to the group. I thought that the best thing was for
me to include everyone in the experience by working on them all
at once. I asked them all to sit still in their chairs while I went to a
nearby building. When I was there, I started to focus on the group.
The energy I can produce when there are that many people in a
room is far greater than when I work in person: it's as if each person's energy is networked into a huge grid. I stayed there for a
while and then returned to the seminar. I was told that people had
started to wriggle in their seats and some of the delegates couldn't
stop moving at all, even to the point where they found their arms
lifting uncontrollably. So despite me being in another building and
there being 300 people, my energy had still managed to affect
them.

I don't usually choose to use my gift in this way, as I don't see the point of showing off with 'party tricks', which I'm sometimes asked to perform. But in this particular situation it was appropriate to do something to quickly show a large group how I could transfer energy. Sometimes you have to be dramatic to get your point across, but usually I save my energy to work in ways that will really make a difference to people's lives.

The positive implication of group and distance healing is that I can reach a wider audience, but the downside is that I can't work on people's beliefs and attitudes as I can do in person. In addition, the strength of energy that's being transmitted during a group session is overpowering for some people and they can find it too much to stand. I find that the best results are achieved through the intimacy of dedicated private sessions. The luxury of time alone with someone allows me to listen to what's going on in their life which may be causing or worsening their condition. It also gives the patient a sense of being special – and the extra lift that comes from feeling cared for and worthy of attention is often a great emotional boost.

Another Dimension

When I connect with someone's energy, I am able to sense things that have happened to them in the past that are relevant to their condition. It's information that I might need to help them heal completely because as well as clearing out the physical energy, I can also work on their mental energy.

I particularly remember one patient who came to me because she felt mentally disturbed. During the diagnosis, I sensed that her uncle had abused her when she was a child. I had to mention this to her because it was critical to her healing that she let out these emotions and recognize what had happened. Although it was painful to bring up, if I hadn't mentioned the abuse, my healing wouldn't have worked so well.

Time does not exist in the body. An event may be in the past, but the memory is still held in the cells, and although it may be hidden deep inside someone, the negative energy has a chain reaction in the body and the effect is always visible somewhere. When I scan someone, I can sense what has happened in their past and also what the future holds for them. To me, it's as if everything is happening in the body now, so I can tell when something needs clearing out. But it's not only during treatments that I am able to see backwards or forwards in time.

Several times in my life I have had premonitions. In 1989 I had a vivid dream in which I was at the top of the telecommunications tower in Sarajevo. I was looking down on my city as it was being bombed. At the time it was a happy and stable place, so I couldn't believe that such destruction would happen. People were running in panic through the beautiful streets below me, and something told me that this was definitely going to happen. It was too real to be a dream – it was as if I was there. I knew that I could do nothing to change the future, so I put this to the back of my mind.

Three years later, in 1992, I received a call from my brother Brano, who was living in Sarajevo. He was crying and told me that war had broken out at home. He must have had an inkling of what was going to happen as he had sent his wife and children to Belgrade two days earlier. He'd sensed something was imminent but hadn't known what. I remembered my dream, and when I saw the news report of the first bombs, the images were just as I had seen in my dream. After I put the phone down, my doors at home blew open. The IRA had planted a bomb at Brent Cross and we had felt the pressure of the blast. It seemed very symbolic, given the news I'd just had.

I had been told many times of my psychic ability, and it has been useful in my work, but at times like this it's harrowing and frightening. The first time I was warned of it was when a lady read my tea leaves in Sarajevo. I was out with a friend and decided to have the reading for fun. It was before I knew I could heal, so I didn't expect anything unusual – just the usual mumbo-jumbo and a bit of a laugh. I expected her to tell me that I'd meet a tall, dark, handsome stranger or something similar. Instead, she told me that I would have the most incredible power and that I'd be able to see into the future. All I could think was 'This must be a joke! Does she really think I'll believe her?' I laughed it off with my friend, and we joked about how I'd been ripped off. Little did I know what was to come.

Even after I'd started to heal, I received messages of what else lay in my future. After I had moved to London, my brother Momo followed with his family; and then my brother Brano, who had returned to Sarajevo after he'd helped me settle in, came back to London for good. Brano, who is an architect, was in his office one day when an Indian man came to visit one of his colleagues. He didn't know Brano at all, but when he saw him, he said, 'I need to meet your sister.' He told Brano that he knew I was a healer, and I was so curious about what he had to say that I agreed to meet him. He said, 'You'll help treat a disease that no one else can help with.' I'm convinced now that he meant that I would help to relieve the trickier symptoms of ME, but at the time, as this was early on in my career, I just took it with a pinch of salt. It's hard to believe things that you're told by a complete stranger, especially when they seem unrealistic! This Indian man went on to tell me that one of the great Tibetan lamas would contact me, and it was at this point that I thought he must be mad. At least I'd been polite and met him, but I really couldn't believe what he was saying. But three years later I did indeed work with a Tibetan lama, Tulku Chime Rinpoche.

Bojan and I had been to Lanzarote for Christmas. We usually stayed for the New Year celebrations, but for some reason I felt like

I had to come back to London. When we got home, there was a message on my answer machine from the Rinpoche's representative in London. It said that he'd heard about me and wanted to meet me. I had to sit down I was so shocked, but it was also an honour to meet him. He asked me to do a blessing for his group in London. I respect the Buddhist religion, but I have always been careful not to align myself with any religious group. I was not brought up to be religious, and I didn't want to close off my treatments to any groups of people. I said this as politely as I could, and the lama asked me, 'What do you believe in?' 'Myself,' I replied. It's true, but it was also the first thing that came into my head. He laughed and said, 'OK. In that case you are more than a Buddhist.'

One of the reasons Tulku Chime had contacted me was because he was losing his sight. I worked closely with him over a period of time, both in London and Tibet, and I helped him regain his sight. We were in contact for five years until he sadly passed away.

My countless experiences of healing people from a distance have led me to believe that time and space aren't as straightforward as we might think. I also know that when we think something's impossible it's often because we haven't yet experienced it – and it's actually a very distinct possibility. I have learned never to say never, and I keep an open mind about everything.

6

UNDERSTANDING AND TREATING ME

Imagine feeling tired, weak, achy and depressed day after day, month after month, and maybe even year after year. That's how many ME patients feel when they come to see me, and they are usually desperate for help. Chronic fatigue syndrome, post-viral fatigue syndrome, 'Yuppie flu' – call it what you like – ME (myalgic encephalomyelitis or encephalopathy) is a controversial disease. It is estimated that the disease affects about 240,000 people in the UK,[1] and although whilst it is most common in people who are between their twenties to early forties, it can develop at any age. The reason it's so controversial is that many people, both within and outside the medical profession, refuse to believe it exists. While the exact cause of ME is yet to be fully understood, it seems that the ME virus, the Epstein-Barr virus, attacks the body when it is weak, for example after a serious bout of flu or glandular fever, and the onset can also come about after a traumatic event, like a bereavement or physical injury.[2]

I first came across ME when I arrived in London. I started to see ME patients and began to notice a pattern. They were in a lot of pain and discomfort, some of them were even in wheelchairs, and

1 Statistic provided by Action for ME. Visit www.afme.org.uk for more information.
2 Information provided by www.cfssupport.netfirms.com.

yet all of their medical tests were negative. They tended to get depressed, partly because the symptoms were very distressing and partly because they were frustrated that doctors found it hard to diagnose or even recognize that they were ill. So they often assumed that there was something mentally wrong with them, and this anxiety didn't help their symptoms. They were fed up of people thinking they were making it up and they started to feel very alienated. I also noticed that most of the sufferers had similar personalities: they tended to be very giving, caring people, like teachers, social workers and healthcare practitioners. They dealt with other people's problems every day and were usually very sensitive to others' feelings. As they became more involved in helping other people, their own energy seemed to drain away.

Another thing I saw was that a common time for people to get ME is during puberty. This is a time of great energetic shift in the body, and sudden surges of hormones can knock the body's immunity. This is often the case for people who experience an early onset of puberty, but as with someone's personality traits, this is never the actual cause of ME. A sensitivity to energy plays a role in the illness, but the disease tends to start when several things are piled on someone at once. By trying to cope with too many things, the body's energy becomes weak; then the immune system gets weaker; and the brain receives less oxygen, which in turn causes many of the symptoms. Contrary to popular belief, as soon as I started treating ME cases, I knew that although glandular fever, bad cases of the flu, inner ear infections, etc. may have been triggers, they were not the root causes.

With so many symptoms to deal with, my first challenge has always been to deal with the anxiety and depression, as it really helps the healing if someone is in a positive frame of mind. The pain caused by other people not believing in this illness is often overlooked, so with some ME cases it can be useful to tell a patient that there is actually something physiologically wrong with them, which of course there is, as this enables them to move on from feeling like a hypochondriac. Since my first case I have seen more than 8,000 ME patients and have also been involved in researching the condition, so I know it's real.

Is It All in the Mind?

One of the reasons why some people still see ME as a psychosomatic illness is because the symptoms are often subjective and intangible. They include extreme tiredness, muscular pain, headaches, depression and problems with memory function and concentration. Chronic fatigue syndrome can be a misleading label and has led to the condition being confused with other undiagnosed conditions, such as hypothyroidism, depression and even some straightforward diet or lifestyle issues. It's no surprise that the condition often attracts cynicism. Another reason why some people don't recognize it as an illness in its own right is because most of us occasionally experience the symptoms, albeit to a lesser degree. Some people believe that this makes it all too easy to self-diagnose, thus making the illness a self-fulfilling prophecy. But whilst the symptoms are relatively intangible to an onlooker, they are real and very distressing to the sufferer. If you've never suffered from it, ME is a difficult condition to relate to or understand, and I find that the best way to grasp an understanding of what people endure is through their own stories.

It all began when I was seven years old. My life was full of exciting things, like school and new friends, but I was always picking up infections. My family was worried that I was always tired and had to miss so much school. Our doctor was as baffled as we were, and he tested me for everything, including leukaemia and glandular fever. After two years I was diagnosed with post-viral syndrome, also known as ME. I was relieved to be diagnosed, but at the same time ME was relatively unknown and people would make thoughtless comments like 'But you don't look ill' and 'Well, you were fine yesterday.'

I had a tonsillectomy in the hope that this would help, but after the operation it became apparent that my tonsils were not the primary cause of my illness. My immune system had completely broken down and my symptoms persisted; chest pains: swollen glands (particularly in my neck, stomach and under my arms), earache, throat pains, stomachache, headache, sore, weak muscles, poor temperature control, fluctuating blood-sugar levels, poor sleep, unbalanced emotions, a feeling of being 'spaced out', muddled mind, candida infections, chronic hiccups, and pins and needles. My symptoms were so bad that I missed school for a year and even climbing the stairs was virtually impossible.

My doctor was extremely supportive and suggested that I see a neurologist. He concluded that my brain seemed to be functioning properly, and we went home none the wiser. In despair, my mother searched for a solution. She saw an article on post-viral syndrome in which Seka was mentioned. After three years of suffering we were willing to try anything.

I vividly remember my first session. My mother and I travelled to North London, and Seka greeted us. She was immaculately dressed and very welcoming. After a chat about my medical history I lay on the bed and Seka made me feel as comfortable as possible.

Seka placed her hands on my forehead and then behind my neck. At first I couldn't feel anything but when she found a weak point in my body, I started to feel intense heat, like a hot-water bottle. It really is hard to describe – it was as if Seka's energy had connected with mine. She fed in positive energy with one hand and removed the negative energy out with the other, making a 'click' sound with her fingers. She moved down my body, and at the very end she brushed her hands down from my head to my feet to remove any last bits of negative energy.

Straight after the treatment I felt peculiar. I felt like someone had thrown away my energy. I was exhausted, and for the rest of the day my symptoms seemed to have got worse. Seka had told me to expect this, but at the time I was sceptical as to whether the treatment had done me more harm than good. But I continued to see her every day that week, and as the week went on I began to feel the results. The good energy that she had given me was really giving me a lift. At that time I had very long, thick hair, and she was of the opinion that much of my energy was being 'zapped' by the energy used to grow my hair, so she recommended that I have my hair cut.

I returned to Seka for a 'booster' treatment, and I then had seven more sessions over three months. Seka continued to balance my energy and also diagnosed a kidney infection, which my doctors hadn't managed to pick up.

My first treatment with Seka was the turning point in my life. I think that the high-dose vitamin C and evening primrose oil that I took helped, but although there was no medical evidence to show that Seka had 'cured' me, I truly believe that without her I would not have made such a successful recovery.

Last year, when I was twenty-one, I was experiencing a difficult time with delayed bereavement and high levels of stress. I decided to return to Seka. It had been twelve years since I'd seen her, but as soon as I entered the room, it was if I'd been treated yesterday. To my amazement, Seka remembered me, not by my medical history but by the weight and thickness of my auburn hair! That one visit was enough to give my energy levels a boost and helped to put my immune system back on the straight and narrow.

I would thoroughly recommend anyone who is experiencing similar difficulties in their life to see Seka. She is an amazing lady who has a tremendous ability to heal people.

Caroline Clarke

When I first started healing, ME was relatively unheard of, but over the years it has become a widely acknowledged disease and the number of sufferers is increasing all the time. I find that this number has increased in direct proportion to the growing stress epidemic. I often see that ME patients have a tendency to use too much mental energy and that they find it hard to draw on their physical energy to support them. This puts enormous stress on the circuitry in the brain, and it's as if the brain becomes overloaded by huge electrical currents, which eventually blows the system. The virus that often underlies ME isn't, therefore, the cause of the illness but is more of a trigger. When the sufferer's energy is particularly low, the trigger is pulled and the virus comes to life. This explanation doesn't prove that the condition is psychosomatic but rather it confirms that stress, particularly mental stress, is a significant catalyst in developing the illness. And so as the world becomes more 'stressful', whatever you want to take that to mean, more people are suffering.

After I had my first few significant successes with ME patients, word of my treatments began to spread through the medical profession and a large number of GPs and consultants found that I had success in relieving symptoms that they were unable to help. Dr Sarah Myhill, one of the UK's ME specialists, heard about me through a consultant paediatrician Dr David Lewis who ran an NHS clinic for ME patients. Dr Myhill admits that her understanding of what I do is restricted by what she calls the 'limited medical model' that she's used to working with, but she agrees that most of the ME patients she's referred to me have experienced a 'quantum leap in improvement'. Her opinion is that I get results and that's all that matters.

Apart from helping me to make some of my strongest relationships with doctors, it was my work with ME patients that attracted the attention of BUPA. They listed me as one of their registered practitioners, and when this happened, it was considered such a significant step towards the recognition of Bio-Energy healing as a reliable healthcare practice that the piece made it onto Sky News.

Looking back, it seems strange to have gained recognition from a medical body for working with a condition that so many medical professionals refuse to recognize. Unfortunately, BUPA couldn't find a way to recognize other practitioners who applied for the same status so, after a while, they decided to no longer recognize healing as one of their supported treatments.

The work I've done with ME patients has also attracted the interest of charities and support groups, mainly because of patients who contacted them after having successful treatments. In 1990 I featured in an article for *InterAction*, the journal published by Action for ME. The piece was written by Leslie Kenton, who was, at the time, the patron of the organization. She opened by saying that she'd had to think long and hard before writing about me because it was 'guaranteed to raise the hackles of self-appointed guardians of "scientific medicine".' However, she decided that the most important thing is that ME sufferers are informed of therapies that may help them, allowing them to come to their own conclusions and decisions. Leslie also said that 'Some chronically ill individuals (not just those suffering from ME) are claiming to have been cured by this treatment, and the majority of those who undergo treatment appear to benefit – many to a significant degree.'

In 1994 I appeared again in the same publication. This second article detailed the relationship I had built with Dr David Lewis. He referred many patients from his NHS clinic to me and described my work as 'close to the phenomenal'. Dr Lewis has found that all of the patients I treated showed a marked improvement, usually within a two-week period, which was sustained. It is satisfying to be recognized and commended by doctors, but the most rewarding thing for me is when patients keep in touch to let me know of their progress.

In 1992, I was diagnosed with myalgic encephalomyelitis. I was suffering from various distressing symptoms, including total exhaustion, twitching, aching muscles, extreme light sensitivity and severe headaches. I was examined by four doctors – my company doctor, the DSS doctor, my own GP and a consultant – and even spent some time in hospital, but all of the tests were negative. Theoretically, there was nothing wrong with me, but I knew there must be. I spent most of the time in my darkened bedroom, exhausted and unable to do very much. I would try to walk to the lounge for my dinner, and on the days when I couldn't, I would crawl instead. My throat muscles had become affected, making it difficult to talk, and I was unable to see friends because my brain wasn't able to understand what people were saying.

Then, luckily, my mum read an article about Seka. I found out that my own consultant at the hospital had referred at least one other patient to her and he wholeheartedly recommended her, whereas he made it clear that he had little time for other alternative treatments. At last it was the day before I was due to meet Seka and I travelled up to London by taxi with my mum and Aunty Cynthia. Quite honestly, I wasn't that hopeful, but I was trying to keep an open mind.

Seka was lovely and she spoke softly, slowly and reassuringly. To begin with, she asked me a few questions and she somehow seemed to know the answers. It was uncanny . . . almost as if she knew me inside out. I wanted to give Seka the list of my ME symptoms, to save us both time, but she wasn't interested. She said these were all 'secondary symptoms' and assured me that once she'd sorted out the main problem, they would all disappear anyway. She knew I'd had a neck injury and my lower back problem; she know all about my allergies and the Raynaud's disease in my hands and feet – and also the fact that I used to work with computers. I don't know how she knew, but she did. Seka then asked me to take off my watch, and she walked towards the door behind me (as though she was about to leave the room). Quite frankly, it was a relief to see the back of her!

Suddenly, though, I felt a tremendous heat on the back of my neck, almost as though someone was standing behind me, holding up an electric fire next to my head. Seka hadn't gone out of the room at all but was standing directly behind me with the palms of her hands a few inches away from my neck. I began to feel very relaxed as the intense heat spread quickly up into my head and then slowly down through the entire length of my body. By now my eyes were watering, my fingers were tingling, and my head had become so hot that beads of sweat were dripping down my forehead. I couldn't understand what was happening. All I knew was that this was the most wonderful feeling I'd ever experienced. It was heaven. She wasn't physically touching me, but I could pinpoint exactly where her hands were from the heat. It wasn't a normal heat . . . it was intense, and although I've tried to describe it as best I can, it really was indescribable.

As I sat there, feeling at peace and so very relaxed with this warm, beautiful feeling running through my body, the most incredible thing happened. I opened my eyes, and for the first time in over two years I was able to look around and actually make sense of what I was look-ing at. My exhaustion had disappeared. My brain was 'alive' just like in the old days. To convince myself I wasn't dreaming, I closed my eyes and opened them again. I started talking to Seka without the slightest hint of pain in my throat. I kept saying, 'I can't believe this. I really can't believe it.' Seka didn't seem at all surprised and said matter-of-factly, 'I've only given you a little bit of energy today – just enough to stop you falling asleep on me! The real healing starts tomorrow.'

She told me that I had an energy blockage in my neck and it was restricting the blood flow to my brain and causing the ME. She went on to say that I'd need four or five treatments on consecutive days and that she'd have me walking within a couple of days. Well, I just sat there in utter disbelief. She just continued to write her notes and casually told me that my particular problem was fairly simple to rectify and that I was 'lucky' in that I only had one energy blockage. I'm not ashamed to admit that I was close to tears – the relief from that crippling exhaustion was just too much for me and I was overcome with emotion.

During my subsequent treatments Seka's confidence and reassurance were so important to me, and once I got home, things began to happen just as she had predicted. I managed to walk around the house several times on the first day, and then each day after that I set myself targets to walk further – to the garden patio, to the garage, to the bird table. Just a week after my last healing session I was able to cycle down to my aunt's house at the end of the road, admittedly free-wheeling a lot of the way, but one week after that I cycled over a mile. A week later I was cycling four miles a day – quite an amazing feat for someone who had been bed-bound for two years!

I still have some way to go, but I hope it won't be too long before I return to my old normal self. However, I'm extremely happy with the way things are. I can do almost anything I want to do (within reason) as long as I pace myself. I recently had a top-up treatment with Seka, four years after she first treated me, and the healing was just as incredible as the previous ones. Since then I've had so much more energy than I've had in recent months. Seka's healing gift is exceptional and unexplainable.

John Bryan

Something that I have found over the years is that many ME sufferers experience a huge list of symptoms and when they come for treatment, they expect me to work directly on these symptoms. My experience of treating these cases has taught me that in true cases of ME there is usually one root problem. There has been a significant amount of research into this, and many doctors agree that the problem is a deficit of oxygen in the brain stem.[3] This deficit leads to malnourishment and, therefore, dysfunction of the nervous and

3 J. Brostoff, D. C. Costa, V. Douli and P. J. Ell, 'Brain Stem Perfusion is Impaired in Patients with Chronic Fatigue Syndrome', *Quarterly Journal of Medicine*, 1995, vol. 88, pp.767–773.

immune systems. Patients of mine, who have had blood tests before and after their treatments, have shown a significant increase in blood oxygen levels, which has reduced their symptoms. Some doctors do acknowledge this deficit in sufferers, but this information has led me to believe, without doubt, that ME is a real condition and not just a figment of the imagination.

Use It or Lose It

With ME cases, once I have started to unblock the energy channels, it's important for the patient to keep the blood flow strong and to keep up the increased oxygen levels. When I treat someone who's suffering with this illness, their oxygen level always rises during treatments. This oxygen deficit causes many of their symptoms: the nervous system can't function to its full ability, so information from the brain to the muscles can only travel slowly; their digestive system doesn't work properly, so they can't get all the goodness from food; and the body can't reach its full potential to do anything. It's critical that these patients keep up their new flow of oxygen because it makes all the difference to their recovery. After charging up a battery, you have to use the energy straight away to make the most of it, and if you don't, the battery can run down again – the body's energy is the same.

I warn my patients on the first day of their treatment that I will expect them to exercise by the third day – even if they have come to me in a wheelchair. I know from experience that it's after the third session of treating someone with ME that their blood circulation speeds up, their oxygen levels really start to rise, and they begin to notice a significant change in their physical strength. By asking people to exercise, I want to take advantage of this significant physical improvement and help them to build up their confidence and belief that they can be well again. When I've 'charged up' my patient, they must make use of the energy soon after I've given it to them, and this has to be done gradually, thus taking them step by step out of the 'comfort zone' of being ill. If they try to do too much too soon, they may feel dizzy, and the last thing I want is for my patients to be afraid or to have their confidence knocked.

Two years after my chronic fatigue syndrome began I tried a number of treatments. Some of them had given me some relief from some of the symptoms, but the basic fatigue problem was getting steadily worse. My daily 'ration' of exercise was two spells of a couple of hundred yards of slow walking, followed by rests. Whenever I exceeded the minimal amount of exercise I'd suffer several days of total physical exhaustion. As someone for whom hill walking had been one of life's great pleasures, this was hard to take.

I arranged to see Seka with little expectation or hope of success. I believed that at the age of fifty-seven I was probably just burnt out.

After the first four days of Seka's treatment I was feeling very disappointed and just as tired and frail as before. After the end of the session, Seka told me firmly that I was to go immediately to Hampstead Heath, which was near to her clinic at the time, for a good walk. Reluctantly, I did as she suggested in the spirit that I would at least show willing, but as soon as it was clear, presumably after a hundred yards or so, that this was yet another unsuccessful treatment, I would return to the car.

After the first hundred yards I felt none of the usual signs that it was time to return and I decided to see if I could manage another hundred yards. And so it went on. That walk on Hampstead Health is fixed in my memory as one of the most astonishing experiences of my life. The more I walked, the better I felt. After an hour of walking at my normal pace I was only just beginning to feel like I'd had enough.

The next day I was naturally very stiff but mentally alert and feeling wonderful. Pretty soon I was working my way through the best mountain walks of North Wales. Seka had only done for me what she has done for so many others, but as far as I was concerned, it was the nearest thing to a miracle I was ever going to see.

Peter Lewis

Rhodri Owen was twenty-two years old when he first came to see me. His ME was so bad he had been bedridden for three years and could barely even talk. I told him on the day of his first treatment that I wanted him to be out of bed by the end of the week – and he looked at me in horror. On the third day I surprised him further by telling him to walk out of the clinic! Rhodri told the *Daily Mail*, 'I thought she was mad, but I walked out of the clinic. I hadn't walked for three months or unaided for three years.' Rhodri's GP, Dr Paul Langley, told the paper that his case was extremely severe and that he had effectively been disabled. I helped Rhodri discover that he was able to do things above and beyond what he believed.

I find that many ME patients are resistant even to a gradual increase in activity. They're used to feeling exhausted and can't believe they'll ever be active again, but that's when I really insist that they start doing something that they used to enjoy. It's vital that they remember what it feels like to move their body.

I got ill gradually during the latter half of 1988; however, it was not until early 1989 that I realized that I was seriously ill and probably had ME. I really couldn't get to work any more, and if I could get there, I was too tired to do anything. I would sometimes think I was fine and then notice that I had my head on the desk while I was thinking this, and that I wasn't actually doing anything!

In the following months I had to stop work, and noticed that I had most of the classic symptoms of ME. Gradually, it became more difficult for me to climb the five steps in my flat, and I got a home help. It became a big venture just to walk slowly to the end of the road. I won't go into all the details here. However, the worst symptoms from my point of view were the brain symptoms; the extreme sensitivity to light and, more seriously, the memory loss – that awful feeling that I just couldn't get my brain to work. At times I couldn't get it to work enough to speak properly. The tiredness, the nausea and the headaches were also hard, and the bad sleep and muscle pain were pretty relentless.

About two years later my symptoms were slightly better but still pretty serious, and I read an article about Seka. Although her treatment sounded exciting I had read about so many different 'magical' treatments that I didn't take a lot of notice. However, soon after this a friend of mine who also had ME came to see me. When I went to the door I couldn't see the dial-a-ride transport for disabled people that she usually came on. I asked her how she got to my place. 'On the bus,' she said. I asked how she got to the bus stop and she said she had walked. I was pretty astonished, and it was then that she told me about her visits to see Seka. After that I felt I had to at least try this treatment. There was nothing to lose and everything to gain.

The first time I went to see Seka for a diagnosis her English wasn't particularly good, so we had only a brief conversation about my health and illness. She then proceeded to move her hands slowly around my body at about ten centimetres distance. It was odd. It was as if she could read my body like a book. She noticed my backache, and when her hands came past my ears, one of my ears started ringing. I asked her about this, and she said, 'Oh, it's just your middle ear – the energy isn't quite right.' I remembered at that point that I had had an operation on my middle ear when I was little. Then her hands came down in front of my chest and one of my breasts started burning a lot. I could feel heat and pain. Seka said that there was nothing seriously wrong there either, but that the energy wasn't right and that she thought that I had a lump in my breast. 'Oh, yes,' I said, 'I've got a cyst in that breast, which I recently had diagnosed.' Seka was quite reassuring that there was nothing badly wrong. Soon after this I felt faint. Seka asked me to lie down. She said that she wouldn't normally give me a treatment with this much energy, but that it was the only way she could do a diagnosis. When she had finished, she said that she thought she could help me and told me to come back the following week every day.

When I left Seka's treatment room and went out onto the street, I felt absolutely fantastic – full of energy and relaxed. I felt good for most of the rest of that day, and a number of people I had never met before commented on how incredibly well I looked!

The next week I went back for my treatments. Each day I lay down while Seka laid her hands on me at different points, working her way down my body. I often felt heat, and sometimes pain, and I also felt relaxed in a way I hadn't done for a long time. Sometimes I felt lots of emotional pain and cried to let it out. I felt safe with Seka, and it felt a relief to get some good rest.

On the third day of treatments Seka told me to go swimming. I had been a great swimmer earlier in my life, often swimming a mile or so. I grew up during my early childhood in Australia, near the ocean, and had learnt to swim well. I went swimming after my treatment with Seka with some trepidation. I can't remember how many lengths I swam, but I went slowly. I was pleased with the fact that I felt good enough to swim again. I was careful not to go too far, and was tired afterwards. I did this again after the fourth treatment and felt encouraged. On the fifth day Seka again told me to go swimming. This time I went to a larger pool, about thirty-three metres, and began to swim breaststoke again. Having had ME for a long time, I was used to looking for energy in my body and finding that I had very little. On this occasion after a few gentle laps I felt myself stretch out and begin to swim properly with bigger stokes. I looked to my body for more energy and was amazed to find that when I called for it, I found it. I began to swim more strongly and felt this wonderful surge of energy. I felt strong. It felt like the kind of energy that I could rely on. This experience was at the time to me like finding a long-lost friend again, and I began to cry. I really felt good swimming. I swam and cried, and when I had done about twenty-two lengths, I suddenly got anxious that I might be overdoing it, so I got out of the pool even though I still felt good swimming. I got dressed feeling exhilarated and still full of energy. I felt so happy. Not only did my body feel energized but my brain felt clear and alive and not fogged up with fatigue. I felt that I had myself back.

In the days that followed I swam too much and sometimes got very tired again; however, I went for a few more treatments with Seka the following week, and she told me that everything was fine, that I didn't need to swim every day, that I could be relaxed about it, but that I must keep swimming regularly. I have done so ever since and now swim between three-quarters of a mile and a mile two or three times a week. Seeing Seka didn't take all my symptoms away immediately, or forever. However, it did get me into a completely different gear. I could begin to build up my physical and mental strength, and my confidence. I have had relapses since, but I am mostly very well. I have gradually got back to work, to singing and to dance lessons. I lead a good and active life. I have weathered some pretty big storms in my life since first being treated by Seka and have found myself astonishingly resilient. I do still sometimes get exhausted, and I sometimes get other symptoms. I have to rest and take care of myself. I go back to see Seka for top-ups every month or two. However, a lot of the time I am well and happy!
Kate Grosser

If you feel that you are at risk of developing ME, if you have suffered or if you are currently suffering from the illness, it's so important that you follow all of the advice that comes later in the Programme for Self-healing (in Chaper 10). By following this, you will learn how to be in tune with your natural frequency so you can see how it is affected by outside influences: you have to acknowledge that a problem exists before we can work with it, so you must begin by recognizing your own energy.

The pain sufferers of ME experience is real; the quality of life they have can be dismal; and the poor treatment they receive is often distressing. I believe that this condition should be taken seriously and that all health practitioners should seek to gain more understanding. Although in my experience there is usually only one root cause for ME for each individual, more often than not it's necessary to take a look at several factors, and one school of thought that I have come to be very familiar with is the effect of environmental and electromagnetic pollution.

7

NEGATIVE RADIATION AND ELECTROMAGNETIC POLLUTION

For most people, home is a secure zone and a place of comfort. We close the door on the outside world and we switch off, relax and regenerate; we assume that we're safe and protected. What I've come to learn, mainly through my contact with ME patients, is that sometimes our homes are not the best place to rest and recuperate and that there are energies in and around the home that can be damaging to our health.

The first kind of energy to watch out for is negative radiation from the Earth. Natural rays penetrate the Earth's surface all the time, and for the most part these rays are harmless. But when these natural rays pass through subterranean water, certain minerals and natural fault lines (cracks in the Earth's strata) their normal frequency becomes distorted and amplified; and this negative radiation can be dangerous to the human body and may cause what's commonly known as, 'geopathic stress'.

The Effect of This Energy on Our Health

The effects of geopathic stress are shown to undermine and weaken human energy. It is thought that this energy interferes with the body's own electrical activity, which, in turn, can distort brain rhythms and interrupt the continual process of cell renewal. This disturbed natural radiation is more harmful to some people than to others, with some people suffering very badly.

At approximately the same time as I moved into my present home I was experiencing a number of stressful events in my life, including bereavement. I didn't sleep very well and constantly felt stressed, but I attributed this to the events happening in my life and to business pressures. I was clearly not well: I picked up numerous colds and other minor ailments and eventually went down with a severe bout of flu. From that point on I just could not get back to anything like reasonable health. I tried everything: antibiotics from my doctor, who also advised me to rest as much as possible, acupuncture, spiritual healing, homeopathy, herbalism, Bach flower remedies, meditation and lots of vitamins, minerals and diet supplements. Many of these things helped – but only temporarily. My symptoms included a sore and burning throat, blocked and sore sinuses, catarrh, a badly congested head, an aching chest together with aches in my neck, back, shoulders, knees and hips, plus general lethargy and extreme tiredness. I would wake up every morning wracked with tension, often having bitten my mouth during my sleep (which was never peaceful) and with aching jaws from grinding my teeth during the night. The strange thing was the longer I stayed in bed, the worse I felt, and the worse I felt, the longer I stayed in bed.

By the following summer I was feeling quite desperate and was wondering whether I would ever feel well again. I spoke to my friend Sarah, who had been treating me for some time with natural remedies. She mentioned that Seka had successfully treated a friend of hers who had ME. After speaking to Sarah's friend, and by now willing to try anything, I made an appointment to see Seka.

She quickly told me that I did not have ME or any other serious illness. She said my problems were caused by extreme stress in my head, neck and shoulders, which was causing a blockage in my body's energy system. She asked whether I had had my house checked for geopathic stress. I had no idea what she was talking about. Seka said that in all the other countries where she has worked there is much more public awareness of geopathic stress than in the UK – in fact, she was appalled by our ignorance. She said that she could cure my condition, so I booked a course of treatment.

Prior to my treatment I would need to have a week to recover from one trip to London. After my treatments, there was a two-week period when I was able to drive up to London and back in a day on ten separate occasions and then work in my office until at least midnight to keep up with my paperwork. I felt, and still feel, better than I have done for at least four years. Seka Nikolic is a truly remarkable lady, and I cannot thank her enough for the help she has given me.

Having had my illness successfully treated, I now had to find the cause. I wrote to the Dulwich Health Society to enquire about geopathic stress. I asked Sarah whether she would come to dowse the house in person. She agreed to come, and she found that damaging energy from the Earth affected many rooms of the house and in my bedroom one extends right across my bed and one metre down from the headboard. I knew this was the cause of my problems.

I slept that night in my spare bedroom – which is unaffected by rays – and for the first time in years I woke up feeling refreshed, without a sore throat and not having bitten my mouth or ground my teeth. I had no feelings of stress and just wanted to get up and enjoy the day ahead. I have been sleeping in my spare bedroom for about two weeks now and the initial benefits have remained the same. I believe I can look forward to even better health in the future.

D.D.

Few people have heard of geopathic stress, but it is becoming a growing, more widely publicized concern. Last year there were a few articles in major British newspapers. One piece told of how a woman who was suffering from breast cancer had stayed with her brother whilst receiving cancer treatment: she was cleared of the disease but on returning home, the disease returned, eventually taking her life. Her daughter began to investigate all the things in and around her home that could have potentially exacerbated her condition, including the electromagnetic fields. A dowser visited her mother's home and found that a stress line ran straight through her mother's bed, potentially having caused, or worsened, her cancer.[1]

Location, Location, Location

When I looked into geopathic stress further, I found out that it is not a recent phenomenon, despite the fact that we are only just becoming aware of it. In 1929 a German doctor, Baron Gustav Freiherr von Pohl, investigated the village of Vilsbiburg in Bavaria in an attempt to find out why this village had an unusually high incidence of cancer. He used divining methods to produce a map of all the significant underground waterways and then matched his map to a map of cancer deaths that had been drawn up by a local medical officer. When the two maps were superimposed, it was found that all the cancer deaths, fifty-four in total, had taken place over the underground streams. Sceptics in the medical community demanded that von Pohl repeat the study, which he did in a different location and with identical results. He went on to conclude that the existence of underground water alone wasn't a decisive factor in determining ill-health, but that the water's speed of flow, the change in seasons and, indeed, the time of day all affected the level of radiation.[2]

In 1990 Christopher MacNaney, of the People's Research Centre

---

1 Ros Weaver 'So you thought you were safe at home . . .', *Observer*, 24 October 2004.
2 David R. Cowan and Rodney Girdlestone *Safe as Houses* (Bath, 1995).

in Cumbria, conducted a study of 750 travellers.[3] He found that the incidence of cancer amongst the traveller community was the lowest in the Western world – a mere 0.6 per cent. This statistic was not a result of a stereotypically healthy lifestyle, as it was noted in the study that travellers smoke, drink and exercise to the same degree as the rest of the nation. Nevertheless, this tiny percentage is in startling comparison with that of the UK as a whole. According to a Cancer Research UK report published in February 2004, more than a third of the population will suffer from the disease at some point in their lives.

The main difference in lifestyle between travellers and the rest of the nation is that travellers are continually on the move, whereas the rest of us seek stability in a fixed location. Any place where we spend a significant proportion of our time is a potential hazard, however, and within our houses the one area where we spend most time is our bed.

If there are harmful lines of radiation rising up from underground streams that are directly below the line of a bed, the occupant may well be spending a third of their life absorbing these frequencies, and given that many of us sleep in similar positions, it is likely that the same part of the body is being exposed continually. To add insult to injury, some coil-sprung mattresses are high conductors of these frequencies, so the type of mattress is also important. Many of us sleep with our heads close to radios and electric alarm clocks, which give off significant amounts of harmful radiation, thereby deeming our bed – a supposed haven of peace and relaxation – to be even more of a danger zone.

We're not all sensitive to these energies to the point of developing an illness, but it is possible for us all to take action. I would advise anyone who thinks they may be in an area of high geopathic stress to have their home looked at, and the most accurate and

3 *Ibid.*

efficient way to detect unhealthy levels of radiation is by getting your home checked by a dowser.

What Is Dowsing?

Dowsing is a term that is most often associated with the divining of water, but dowsers can also measure naturally occurring and man-made magnetic fields. Some dowsers use equipment, but most dowsing is done with dowsing rods. The rods appear to move on their own, but it's the energy of the dowser that shifts. The energy change, which is usually very small, moves up the dowser's legs and up the body into the hands, where the rod picks it up and magnifies it.

I am able to dowse, as are many people who are sensitive to energy, but it drains me because I'm not a transformer for that kind of energy. I prefer to check for energy with my hands, and whenever I move somewhere new, I always do a quick check. I also check every treatment room I use to make sure the energy is neither too still nor too turbulent. Many people can sense energy as soon as they walk into a room. To dowse, you need to be very relaxed, but the key thing is to trust your intuition and clear your mind. If you're looking to move to a new house, see if you can forget the price, location and so on for a moment to see how you feel about a place – your sense will tell you a lot.

Dowsing isn't generally recognized in the UK, but in many other European countries it is widely accepted. In Russia, dowsing is taught as a science in its own right, and many dowsers there are qualified doctors, engineers and scientists. In Poland, it is soon to become the law that certain types of buildings can only be erected following a dowsing test by a state-registered inspector.[4] Germany

4 Alfred Riggs.

is also home to many dowsing experts, and Professor Hans-Dieter Betz, Professor of Physics at Munich University, has led a research study that looked at the ability of dowsers to locate underground drinkable water in ten different countries. It was found that even in difficult geological conditions, the dowsers had a 96 per cent success rate, often taking under an hour to complete the task. In comparison, geohydrologists who were given the same task had a 21 per cent success rate and took two months to evaluate a site.[5]

What Does This Mean for You?

This information does *not* mean that geopathic stress definitely causes illness. It's also important to clarify that this theory does not deem that all illness is caused by geopathic stress. These findings do show, however, that geopathic stress is one of the factors that can cause disease and that by weakening the body, it provides a fertile ground in which ill health can flourish.

The most common symptoms of geopathic stress are resistance to conventional or complementary therapy, exhaustion, depressed mood, anxiety, insomnia, allergies, cramps, grinding of teeth, headaches, a fuzzy head and an excessive feeling of cold. The illnesses that are most likely thought to be caused by geopathic-induced immune problems are cancer, ME and MS.

The reason that geopathic stress can lead to illness is because it depresses the immune system and therefore the body's ability to fight disease. The body does most of its regeneration and repair work on cells whilst we are sleeping, so if we are sleeping in an area that is rich with unhealthy energies, the immune system can't work to full capacity.

5 Hans-Dieter Betz, Water Dowsing in Arid Regions: Report on a Ten-year German Government Project', *Journal of Scientific Exploration*, Stanford University, California, 1995.

Electromagnetic Pollution

We have been blessed in many ways by the developments of technology and science, but it turns out that we are also cursed by them. Whilst we have to watch out for the Earth's energies, another kind of energy we need to be aware of is electromagnetic energy that is a by-product of modern life. This is often called electromagnetic pollution.

Electricity is a major power source for the world, and with the advent of new gadgets, we are continually adding to the electromagnetic web that cloaks the Earth. It's commonly believed that energy created by modern technologies contributes to electromagnetic pollution, and this includes energy from electricity pylons, transformers, telecommunications towers, radio towers and even mobile phones. In addition to this, lighting, heating, computers, domestic appliances, stereos, televisions, railways, telecommunications and even exercise equipment all have live electrical wiring that radiates harmful magnetic fields into our environment.

Because of their transmission systems and their dominance in our lives, radio and television waves fill our atmosphere to the extent that they can be picked up in almost any place on the planet, no matter how remote it is. This makes for a convenient life, but our bodies have yet to evolve to deal with the resultant magnitude of radiation. This is becoming a growing concern, hence the need for the UK's National Radiological Protection Board, which investigates the effect of radiation on human health.

In 2004 a newspaper ran a piece entitled 'Power lines double risk of cancer in children'.[6] There have been claims that research like this has been suppressed by the Department of Health. This article made very clear the controversy surrounding the issue.

6 Charles Arthur, 'Power lines double risk of cancer in children', *Independent*, Saturday, 30 October 2004.

Some studies have concluded that the risk of electromagnetic fields causing cancer are tiny, but regardless of the size of the risk, surely the public has a right to be made aware of any information like this. These kinds of findings have potentially very far-reaching effects for society, and Maureen Ashby, the President of the Trentham Environmental Association Campaign told the paper, 'The Government should act now. We aren't prepared to wait ten years while they dither.'

Many people are convinced of the effect of electromagnetic pollution on health. The best we can do is seek help from a dowser, many of whom are skilled and accurate in their analyses of both natural and man-made energies. One of the most well-known and respected men in this profession is Alfred Riggs.

The Effect of These Energies on ME

Alf is someone with whom I work very closely. He used to be the head of science and technology for the British Society's Earth Energies Group and director of Sanaway, the bio-medical specialist. He is now a full-time dowser, or radiethesist, as he prefers to call himself. The word radiethesist, comes from the root words for radiation and perception and is most often used in the UK in the medical arena. Alf became involved in his current field of work in the 1960s when he set out to discover what caused disease. As a result of his research, he discovered that geopathic stress and electromagnetic pollution have a significant effect on health. Alf now devotes all of his time to checking homes and offices for potentially harmful radiation.

I first got to know Alf when he sent me one of his ME patients. Whilst he was able to clear his clients' homes, he wasn't in a position to heal them. Conversely, as I gained experience with ME patients, I found that there was no point treating these patients if

they continued to live in a house which was dangerously affected by these energies, so after our first successful case together, Alf and I have continued to refer patients to each other.

I had seen an Action for ME article about Seka and had heard of others who had been healed of ME. Having suffered for nearly a decade, I decided to see Seka.

Day 1

Seka started by passing her hands over my aura and in only a few minutes told me three conditions that I knew I had and others besides. Those directly relating to ME were: reduced blood flow to the right side of the brain, reduced blood flow to the brain stem and heart palpitations caused by lack of blood to the brain stem – not a major heart problem. She also told me of Alf Riggs' research and showed me results of his home visits, which showed correlations between his findings and cases of cancer and ME. Seka advised me to contact Alf, and I knew that radiation/electromagnetic effects in my home could undo her work.

Day 2

Treatment started. Seka sat behind my head and cradled the back of it in her lovely warm, firm hands. Then she moved around the head and, later, down the body, ignoring my limbs until the end. After each cradling, she held one hand on me whilst she shook the other hand, making a clicking sound. One hand was feeding in energy whilst the other released it with the noise of static electricity. At organs that needed healing, she spent more time, and the organ, not the skin, glowed with heat in response. She told me to rest and to try not to do too much for the rest of the day. I slept for two hours that afternoon.

Day 3

I was whacked! I could hardly sit up in the waiting room. The procedure was the same as on the first day. I was much better than the day before, although I went home to rest as usual.

Day 4

Seka told me that I could start to be more active. I had also had head and chest pains from a cold that had started. She treated this too. I needed painkillers, but Seka said, 'it will go.' It did – by the time I'd had lunch at the bottom of Regent Street. I went on to spend two hours shopping in Oxford Street and walked to Marble Arch tube station.

Day 5

Seka told me the healing would continue for another fortnight and asked me to write to tell her how I was in six weeks' time. I needed to start to do more exercise – swimming, walking or cycling. She said I might need three days' booster treatments. I travelled back up North, glad to meet friendly folk on the homeward train. London is so isolating!

End of week 2

I borrowed my daughter's crash helmet and bike and cycled up the road (about half a mile). You should have seen folk's amazement and laughter! After a week I cycled down to the bottom of the hill and back home. I have now done this most days and have doubled my exercise.

I also saw Alf Riggs on Seka's advice. I met him at the station. I thought he was a very quiet man, having had a brief phone conversation with him. But from the minute we got in the car he was a mine of information for the rest of the day.

After measuring the geopathic stress in our house, his verdict was that we have an underground stream, the edge of which passes diagonally across the house, crossing my daughter's bed. She too has ME and he said 'She'll never get better if she sleeps there.' Our radios were too close to our heads when we were in bed – he suggested moving them out of reach from the bed. He showed us which mattresses were the safest. Even two identical ones gave different readings, and the safest was the old one that sags! My daughter has seen significant changes after only six weeks of changing bed.

Harriet

Alf has worked with over three thousand cases of ME in more than twenty countries. His work has led him to conclude that ME is primarily a bioelectric problem. He also claims that the Earth's energy field interacts with oestrogen and alters the messages that are then sent along the body's electrical system, which he believes explains why ME is a predominantly female illness.[7]

Despite all this evidence, ME continues to divide the orthodox medical profession and the scientific community, although some doctors are sitting up and taking note.

I have read about Seka's work, and one of my patients has been substantially helped by her. Seka has treated over 1,900 patients with CFS and tells me that 90 per cent do well. Such is her reputation that she is booked up with work many months ahead. However, what is particularly interesting to me is that the very symptoms that she is best at treating (brain fog, fatigue, malaise) are the ones that remain in my 'failures'. Her work is done in conjunction with Mr Alf Riggs, who visits the patient's home and checks it for geopathic stress and electromagnetic pollution.

Dr Sarah Myhill[8]

7 For more information on dowsing and geopathic stress, visit the British Society of Dowsers' website on www.britishdowsers.org, Alfred Riggs' website, www.alfredriggs.com, or Roy Riggs' site, www.royriggs.co.uk.

8 Dr Myhill's website, www.drmyhill.co.uk, contains a wealth of information on ME. She has put this information together into a book, which can be ordered via her site.

But the connection of geopathic stress and electromagnetic pollution to disease is sadly not limited to ME. Alf claims that all the cases of multiple sclerosis that he's worked with have been located in areas of stress. He also said that he has seen many cases of geopathic-induced cancer and claims that he has yet to work with a person suffering from chronic lymphoid leukaemia who isn't living in the presence of dangerous radiation.

Alf has also worked with a German dowser, Kurt Weinburg, on behalf of a cancer clinic. The clinic gave them a list of people's addresses and asked them to check their beds and report back with their findings including which beds belonged to the cancer sufferers and even what kind of cancer they had. For example, in one house there were five beds, and both Alf and his colleague found only one problem bed and predicted, from where they found the lines of energy, cancer of the throat. The man who slept there did indeed have cancer of the throat, and his first wife, who had slept in that same position, had died of the same cancer. I recommend all of my patients to Alf, and those who use him are always astounded at how accurately he can pinpoint the problem.

Another doctor with whom Alf worked very closely was the late Dr Hans Alfred Nieper. Nieper was a world-renowned cancer specialist and president of the German Society of Oncology. He is said to have been consulted by several famous people, including Yul Brynner and Ronald Reagan. Dr Nieper stated that over 70 per cent of all his cancer patients and about 75 per cent of his MS patients were geopathically stressed.[9]

So we can see that several doctors and scientists have concluded through years of research that we are indeed affected by these radiations and that location is a key determinant in the occurrence of certain diseases. In addition, one doctor, Dr Robert Jacobs, believes that the main negative effect of geopathic stress is that it stops

9 Dr Joseph Mercola, 'Geopathic Stress', taken from the website www.mercola.com.

patients from recovering. He claims that it seems to make a patient resistant to the action of almost all types of therapy: 'When patients tell me that they have already seen two homeopaths, an acupuncturist and three Harley Street consultants, none of whom could get them better, I find that they are usually suffering from geopathic stress. I suspect that geopathic stress is the only reason for natural remedies to fail. If a patient does not respond to correctly administered remedies and assuming that the disease is potentially treatable, one usually finds that they are suffering from geopathic stress.'[10] This is because these rogue energies disrupt the body's electrical system – the very system that determines the rate and power of healing in the body

What Does the Future Hold?

We are becoming more aware of our environment, but other countries, such as Australia, Austria, Germany and Russia, are much more active in their research of geopathic stress than we are in the UK. Research into geopathic stress needs to bring together the subjects of astronomy, physics, biochemistry and physiology in order to be a truly holistic study. Dr Eugene Melnikov, a Russian geologist, has carried out research with a multidisciplinary team of scientists. They have concluded that earth radiation causes biological damage to humans, animals and plants. It seems that by using scientists from different disciplines, Melnikov has managed to get a clear picture of the situation.[11] Alf Riggs is also so confident in his conclusions that he regularly offers to demonstrate his

10 Dr Robert Jacobs, MRCS, LRCP, 'Geopathic Stress', taken from the website www.wholisticresearch.com.
11 Elizabeth Brown, *Environmental Energies – The Missing Piece of the Jigsaw?* taken from an interview conducted by James Whale and available on the website www.whale.to.

findings in a double-blind test environment to any respected university, but no one has yet taken him up on his offer.

Geopathic stress remains a mystery to many because it is relatively intangible. It is in our nature as human beings to seek tangible evidence of causes and symptoms, but that said, we live, unquestioningly, with a number of intangible phenomena. We cannot touch negative emotions, such as anger and fear, and we cannot see scientific phenomena, such as radio waves and X-rays, but we know they exist and we allow these things to infiltrate and disturb our everyday existence. Geopathic stress and electromagnetic pollution will remain a mystery until the medical world at large is prepared to accept that our biological framework is affected at a cellular level by electromagnetic frequencies.

I was suffering from ME and had been treated by Seka. A few years after seeing her I read an article in one of the local papers and my mind flashed back to something Seka had said. The article was about geopathic stress and a local dowsing society that was looking for a new member. I thought I might as well give the chap a call and ask him if he'd mind dowsing my bungalow.

Within an hour he was walking down my drive with a dowsing rod in his hand. He told me that a geopathic stress line was running through the length of the bungalow. As I followed him around, both of us watching the rod for any slight movement, the rod suddenly swung violently to the left. Yes, he'd discovered another geopathic stress line, this one crossing the first one at a ninety-degree angle directly under my bed. The second line was running in a straight line through my bedroom and along through Mum's room. Looking quite concerned now, he said, 'One's bad enough, but two crossing each other . . .' He took a deep intake of breath. The dowser went on to tell me of the negative effects, just as Seka had done all that time ago.

In addition to the geopathic stress lines, there was also a curry line, a particular kind of radiation line, running diagonally across them. Apparently, this was the 'worst combination you could get', and he advised me to sleep in another room or, better still, move house.

Being highly sceptical, I still wasn't totally convinced, despite the amazing coincidences. But since that day I have slept in the lounge (the only room not affected) and I have to say I've never slept so well in my life. I'm finally free of the insomnia that plagued me for years. I sleep like a log and wake up feeling completely refreshed each morning.

So, having lived for several years in close proximity to a small electricity sub-station and having worked for many years a short distance from overhead power lines as well as a large, 132 kV sub station, I feel that my body has had excessive amounts of exposure to the harmful effects of electromagnetic radiation. I think my immune system was affected by all of these things and that something else, perhaps my neck injury, caused the energy blockage that triggered the ME.

J.B.

What Are the Signs of Geopathic Stress?

Many people who suffer illness at the hands of electromagnetic radiation have experienced significant improvement in their symptoms by making a few simple changes to their home. Here's some advice for you should you feel that you'd benefit from it. There are a number of signs that you or your home may be affected by geopathic stress:

Common Symptoms of Geopathic Stress That You Could Be Suffering From

- You have any serious illness.

- Your illness isn't responding to appropriate treatment.

- You've tried a number of different therapies – conventional and complementary – without success.

- Your symptoms clear up or improve when you are away from home, for example on holiday.

- You became ill shortly after moving house.

- Your home has never felt comfortable and you felt ill at ease as soon as you moved in.

- You wake up feeling groggy in the mornings, even when you've had enough sleep.

Signs of Geopathic Stress in the Home

- There is mould in the house.

- There is a lot of lichen or moss growing on the roof, walls, or lawn – these plants thrive in areas of geopathic stress. Other plants include oak, fir, elderberry, peach and cherry trees and mistletoe.

- Your house may have a problem with ants, wasps or bees, as they are attracted to these energies.

- There are cracks in walls, driveways, paving slabs and roads – this may be a sign that your home is on a geological fault line.

- There are trees that have split in two or that have large, knobbly or strange growths. If the branches look as if they're trying to get out of the way of something, they probably are.

- Your close neighbours are in poor health.

- There are springs or wells nearby.

- Previous occupants of the house were ill.

- Animals are sensitive to geopathic stress. Horses, dogs, cows, sheep, pigs and mice would not willingly sit over areas of geopathic stress, so if the dog has a favourite spot in your house, it's safe! On the contrary, cats are attracted to geopathic stress so avoid sleeping or sitting for long periods anywhere that your cat likes to settle.

If you or your home have any of the above symptoms, it doesn't necessarily mean you are ill or in danger. It does mean that you should look at your health and see if you can find any correlation with what you've read here. If you think you can, then contact a reputable dowser or the British Society of Dowsers.

What Can You Do About Electromagnetic Pollution?

There are some things you can do straight away to reduce the electromagnetic frequencies in your home:

- Use your mobile phone only when you have to or for quick calls; otherwise use a landline.

- Protect yourself from your computer with a protective screen. These are available from most computer hardware stores.

- Avoid sitting with electric cables under your chair or desk.

- Where possible, avoid spending any time near power stations.

- Remove electrical equipment from the bedroom, including radio-alarm clocks, hairdryers, televisions, electric blankets, mobile phones, computers and cordless digital telephone bases.

- Set up your digital telephone base and wireless Internet connection in a part of the house where you don't spend much time.

- Turn off your broadband when you're not using it, and don't get a wireless network unless you really have to.

- If you can, switch to an analogue phone – you can buy cordless ones.

- Remove electrical toys e.g. train sets from your children's bedrooms.

- Do not sleep on a coil-sprung mattress.

- Do not sleep on magnetic pillows or mattresses.

- Only use baby monitors when you absolutely have to.

Sometimes when I make suggestions like these to people, they find that they are so used to the convenience of electrical appliances or they're in the habit of keeping things where they are that they don't want to make any changes. We always have a choice over what we do, and given the knowledge I've learned about geopathic stress, I would strongly recommend that anyone who thinks they may be at risk makes these relatively small changes for the sake of their health.

8

THE IMPACT OF EMOTIONS

We are emotional beings – it's one of the things that makes us human, and most people accept that our health is affected by our feelings. Unfortunately, these are not the only emotions that influence how we feel: we are also affected by the emotions of other people. But before we look at how we can protect ourselves from the moods of others, let's see how we can manage ourselves.

I've seen from living in different countries and from treating patients from different cultures that each of us is capable of showing and hiding our emotions to varying degrees, but what most of us tend to do, regardless of our culture, is show happy emotions – like love, excitement, confidence, joy – and hide the emotions that we think are a sign of weakness – such as anger, sadness, fear and embarrassment. We can probably get away with blocking our emotions for a short while, but eventually the pressure of suppressing them becomes too much and the emotions will either explode or implode, having a knock-on effect on our health.

The Frequency of Emotions

Each emotion has its own frequency. Negative emotions, like sadness, anger, anxiety and fear, vibrate at a low level, and positive ones, like excitement, happiness and love, resonate at higher frequencies. We experience the changing frequencies of these emotions through very real physical shifts: the uplifting emotions, such as joy, exhilaration and love, make us feel light and energetic, but the negative ones, like worry, depression, grief and fear, make us feel heavy and lifeless. Think about how you feel when you have different moods. Can you remember the contrast both in your body and your mind? These energetic frequencies can either make us healthier or make us unwell – and there's no prize for guessing which way around it is!

We can't avoid feeling negative emotions, but we can learn to be sensitive to how our mood changes and how our energy changes accordingly. By becoming aware of our own natural frequency, we can learn to sense when something isn't right for us and avoid it. By learning to regulate the shifts in our energy, we take the most basic step in maintaining our mental and physical health.

If you are interested in healing yourself, it's important to start by noticing how emotions feel in your body. You'll soon begin to realize whether they're having a positive or negative impact on your health, and once you've done that, you can start to control how you feel, so that your health can flourish.

We have a choice over our emotions. Even if we become upset because of something that's outside of our control, we are able to choose how we react. I realize that there are times when it's natural and healthy to have a negative feeling, for example when we are grieving, but a lot of the time we hold on to our emotions for way too long.

Think back to a time when you were frustrated. It may have been over something like a delayed train or a failed promise. How long did you allow yourself to feel frustrated? What did that feeling do for you? What impact do you think that had on your body?

Looking back, what other emotion could you have picked that would have been more helpful or uplifting?

I hope that you can see from this quick, simple exercise how we are affected by our emotions – and also how we really can control them to make ourselves feel better. Now let's look at other people's emotions.

What About Other People?

We can tell how someone is feeling by the obvious things, like what they say, how they move and the expression on their face, but we also communicate how we feel through our energy. I don't know if you've ever called someone and before they have even spoken, you know that something is wrong. Or you walk into a room and within a split second you can feel the atmosphere. You haven't had enough time to look around or read the situation – you just know that something is amiss. We can also sense when someone is thinking about us. Have you ever telephoned someone just as they were about to ring you? Or received an email from a friend who you dreamt about the night before? Can you sense when someone is looking at you across a room? And can you ever tell what someone else is thinking? When we experience situations like these, it seems that there is more at play than just coincidence: we are experiencing an energetic connection with another person. Phrases such as 'We're on the same wavelength', 'You're so in tune with each other', 'The atmosphere was electric', 'He sent shivers down my spine', 'They got a good feeling about it' or, 'I feel that we're in sync' are common in our language, but we don't often think about what they really mean. There's no doubt that we are affected by the thoughts and emotions of other people, and these, in turn, can affect our health.

When the late Princess of Wales passed away, I remember how

the country was caught up in a whirl of sadness. I was touched because I had had the honour of meeting Diana, but even people who had never met her or those who claimed they didn't care found themselves caught up in the tide of grief that swept over the world. But it's not just grief that's infectious: any kind of strong atmosphere can be contagious. My son, Bojan, plays in a band, and whenever I go to one of his gigs, I can see how the crowd gets lifted by the music. There's something in the energy of the sound that makes people feel good. You also see how energy gets communicated at other events, like football matches, political demonstrations, weddings and funerals. Events like these are so full of passion that it's easy to become overwhelmed by them. Some psychologists say that the phenomenon of 'crowd behaviour' is because of 'de-individuation' or a feeling of weakened responsibility. This means that people feel safer in a group and so they're more expressive than they would usually be.[1] Others say that it boils down to a mathematical formula.[2] These theories may be true to a certain extent, but I believe that emotions are contagious because of the spreading and sharing of energy.

We Can't Help It

I was having lunch with a friend the other day and we were sitting next to two elderly ladies. They must have been well in to their eighties, and they were dressed up in smart suits with glamorous handbags and red lipstick. From the minute we sat down we could tell they were really enjoying each other's company. We couldn't hear what they were saying, but they gave off a powerful vibrancy.

1 William F. Ogburn and Meyer F. Nimkoff, *A Handbook of Sociology* (London, 1964).
2 G. K. Still, 'New Insights into Crowd Behaviour – It's Fractal', *Focus*, November 1994.

Just as we were about to leave, we started chatting to them, and they were so much fun! We laughed and joked for only a few minutes, but I left the restaurant and went back to work feeling invigorated and happier than I had when I sat down. We had exchanged a very positive energy.

Unfortunately, we don't always choose the energy that's around us. We may attend a demonstration, concert or wedding because we want to, but sometimes we have little choice over who we spend our time with or the situations that we get involved in. We don't choose who we sit next to on the train or bus; we have little choice over who we meet at work; and we have to interact with lots of people on a daily basis – the bus conductor, the shop assistant, the postman, the delivery boy, a waitress, our clients and people we meet at parties. So a lot of the energy we come into contact with is not through choice.

Other people's energy field affects us like we're affected by the weather. If it's a humid day, we feel hot and sticky; if it's cold, we feel chilly; and if it's raining, we get wet – we can't help but be affected by the atmosphere and temperature, and it's the same with human 'atmosphere'. So if we're talking to someone or in the same room as them, we take on some of their energy. Their vibration is transmitted invisibly through the air, and we unconsciously tune in to it like we can tune in to radio waves. Think about some specific examples. We may be drawn to a piece of music, or we can flinch if a song doesn't sit well with us. We all know people who make us feel calm and people whose enthusiasm is catching. We've all met someone with whom we immediately feel at ease, and we've all come across people who make us bristle. As soon as we meet someone we exchange energy, and it's the same with places and things: some rooms and buildings feel friendly and welcoming, and others make our hair stand on end. One of my favourite places is Lanzarote. The mountains and the sea give off the perfect frequency for me to relax, which is the main reason why I keep going back there.

Why Does This Happen?

Remember back to what I said about energy: everything is made up of energy. Every person, object, place and sound gives off a vibration, and our energetic antennae tune in to the frequencies that surround us. Sometimes those frequencies feel good, and sometimes they don't. We are affected by energetic fields all the time, and as well as judging energy with our five senses, we use our sixth sense to suss them out. We instinctively know whether an external energy vibrates at a compatible frequency by whether we feel safe and comfortable. Sometimes we do this consciously, but most of the time we're unaware of it. We can't explain why we're drawn to certain things and people – all we know is that they make us feel good. If we vibrate at a frequency that is right for us, then we feel stronger and more vibrant and this has a positive effect on our health. But as you already know, our health can be negatively affected too.

I recently treated a lady who had married a deeply religious man. She had entered into her marriage unaware of how she would have to adjust to such a devout way of life, and she hadn't really thought about what would be expected of her. Once she was married, she was shocked at some of the practices and responsibilities that she had to take on, but she had no choice. She felt so alienated that she had started to lose her normal mental faculties. She told me that she would go to pick up her children from school and she couldn't tell one child from another. She couldn't even recognize her own children. She saw things completely differently to everyone else – she was so caught up in her own problems that she had literally lost sight of the world around her.

During her treatments I helped her adjust her view of the world, and she started to get back in touch with reality. I helped her reconnect with her own identity so she could regain a sense of herself. But I knew that it was going to be a challenge for her to maintain this balanced state when she was back in her day-to-day environment.

We all have our own personal space – the space that's taken up by our electromagnetic energy field, or aura. Most of us can't see these fields, but we can all feel them, especially when we get too close to something that makes us feel uneasy. For me, one of the most extreme examples is when I go into a hospital. Because of the intense sick energy, I immediately feel drained. This strong energy really throws my own energy, and by interacting with fields like this, my natural frequency can become de-tuned, like when one radio signal interferes with another.

As I have developed my sensitivity to energy, I have also developed ways to protect myself from negative energy. This energy might come from something I'm reading or watching on television or from someone I'm speaking to. I can tell when a suggestion can affect my own decisions or behaviours in the wrong way, and I start to distance myself from it. If I'm reading, I can still see the words but I don't feel attached to them, and if someone's talking, their voice starts to fade, as if I'm outside the situation. By detaching myself in this way, I protect myself not only from the content of what's said but from its energy as well. For example, if someone tells you that you look unwell and you accept what they say, your energy and health will change in a second. But once you start to recognize the power of suggestion, you begin protecting yourself. Knowledge and awareness are forms of protection, and the more we know about our body, health and energy, the stronger we become.

The Scientific Explanation

Whenever I come across an idea that isn't widely accepted, I look for a scientific explanation of what's going on. I like the rational aspect of science, and it also helps me to explain things to other people. It's made a difference to my patients that I can help them to understand Bio-Energy by drawing parallels with electricity and radio signals: it puts what is a relatively unfamiliar concept into the realms of daily life, which makes it much easier to grasp. So what does science have to say about invisible communication?

You would think that two objects that are miles apart would have no connection with each other, but the basic laws of physics tell us differently. Even though they're 93 million miles apart, the Earth and the Sun are connected by an electromagnetic energy field, which we know as gravity. We can't see it, but we know it exists. We feel the effect of gravity every day, and it holds us to the ground, makes us drop things and causes us to fall down. Another familiar thing that works through an invisible communication system is the battery-operated transistor radio. It stands alone from any other object, yet it picks up and connects with radio frequencies that are given off by transmitting devices. And I'm sure you either have or know someone who has a mobile phone. These give us an invisible connection with all corners of the world, and we definitely take them for granted. So you can see that we live inside a web of energy fields, all of which communicate and interact with each other.

What Has This Got to Do With You?

All things in the universe are interconnected, so when one thing changes, everything else around it changes. If a stone is thrown into a pond, the ripples affect the water in the pond as well as all the plants, animals, boats and people in it. As the ripple extends further out, it becomes subtler until you can barely feel it, but it's still there.

It's easy to understand this physical interconnection of energy, but energetic communication is happening all the time from person to person, and whether you realize it or not, you experience it every day. Call it what you like – energy, mood, electromagnetic field or aura – our brains transmit these waves of energy, and they broadcast our frequency into the atmosphere. Scientists have researched this way of communicating, and they're starting to use this invisible energy to help people who can't communicate by speaking.

Brain cells communicate by producing tiny electrical impulses. These impulses are sent through the nervous system to tell parts of the body to act or react. Scientists can now capture these currents by placing electrodes on the scalp, which allow them to input these signals into a computer where the person's thoughts can be translated into messages. This has led to the development of brain–computer interface (BCI) systems that allow someone to communicate without having to speak or move.[3] This is a fantastic development for anyone who is paralysed but who has retained brain function. One American research team claims that we will soon be able to control artificial limbs and robots just by thinking about it. So far, the research has proved to be successful: a quadriplegic man has been able to move a computer cursor, and a monkey has moved a robotic arm – both with the power of thought alone.[4] These findings are not only being used to bring about advances in the medical arena; a video game has also been developed in which the player wears a headset that analyses all their

3 Linda Lim, 'Tapping Brain Waves', *Innovation*, vol. 5, issue 1.
4 Carl Zimmer, 'Mind Over Machine', *Popular Science*, February 2004.

thoughts, allowing them to control their character's actions just by thinking about them. These developments are just a few examples of the research that is being undertaken using the radio waves that we emit from our brains.

These technological advances prove that thought and emotions can be transmitted as energy. Whilst these projects show that these waves can be detected externally, by computers, I strongly believe that humans are also able to pick up on these energies directly. We've seen that this discovery can be used to help people who have neurological problems, but it can also help us learn how to protect ourselves and take care of our health: if we know what's happening, we can stop it. For a long time I have known how significantly we are affected by energies around us, and I have witnessed this in many of my patients.

I treated a girl who was suffering very badly from anorexia nervosa. She was in her early twenties and was still living with her parents. They came with her to the first appointment, and I could see that they had a very powerful and controlling effect on their daughter's behaviour. When they came into my room, I immediately felt uneasy, as if there was a cloud of tension around them. This negative, heavy vibration was stifling the young girl's energy, which caused her natural frequency to shift, and as a result, she was eating unnaturally. I worked on her energy field, and I also encouraged her to become more independent. She needed to distance herself from the damaging energy of her family so that the changes I'd helped her make could last.

There's no point me treating someone if they just return to their old ways. It's the same with any change we make; we need to make it a habit for it to last. If we eat more healthily and exercise, we will lose weight, but if we then go back to our old habits of stuffing ourselves and sitting around, the weight will come back. If someone drinks too much and has damaged their liver, they can help cure themselves by giving up alcohol, but if they start drinking heavily again, they will reverse the good work. The same rule applies to the energies around us, whether they're from people, places or thoughts; if we remove ourselves from the negative energy, our healthy changes will last, and we have to either stay away from them or become immune to them. But there are times when it can be hard to do this.

It's a Family Affair

Most of us spend our early years surrounded by our families. We usually take on our parents' beliefs and behaviours, and we become so used to their frequencies that we don't notice if they're unhealthy for us. Culture, religion, habits and relationships – all of these things seem like second nature to us, and we don't often question them. My mother and father had solid, balanced opinions on health, education and family, so I'm lucky to have adopted these beliefs, but not everyone is so fortunate. Most parents want what's best for their children, but sometimes they don't realize what that is. If you think that you receive unhealthy energy from your family or anyone else, you don't have to totally cut yourself off – you just have to learn to be your own person.

My skin problem began when I was fourteen. In fact, I can remember the first day I experienced facial acne like it was yesterday: I went to bed on Friday night with a face clear of spots and woke up the following morning with a red, swollen lump on the left-hand side of my chin. It was as painful as it looked, and I was at a total loss as to how to deal with it. My father drove me to the hair salon where I worked on a Saturday and just kept saying how ugly it was and how it should be a lesson to me to not get run down and to have early nights. But I was already doing all that. As usual, my parents were controlling everything

I did – not giving me any choices or the chance to grow up as my own person.

This lump took weeks to go. Just as it was about to fade, another lump took its place. And this was how it was for the next few years. At the weekends I could at least try to hide my skin with make-up, but make-up wasn't allowed at school, so I had to suffer the teasing. At night I would carefully cleanse my skin, and I tried all the creams on the market. Nothing worked. This went on for years. I felt totally alone, and my confidence and self-esteem were shattered. My parents told me that it was my fault and gave me no support at all.

When I went to university, I met a girl who suffered from acne too. She told me in confidence that if I went to see my GP, he would be able to prescribe me with antibiotics, which would improve the problem. I followed her advice. They actually did start to help, but at a cost: I remember being at home on holiday and my mother telling me to stop the tablets as they were making my skin smell unpleasant – the smell was coming through my pores. I was shattered.

Just before my final exams, my father made an appointment for me to see a dermatologist but this was totally impractical – the dermatologist was hard to get to on public transport (my only option), and with only a few weeks before my exams, every day was valuable revision time. Much to my father's disgust, I cancelled the appointment.

When I left university, I stopped the antibiotics and the problem got worse. At my first job I met another acne sufferer. She told me about a new drug on the market. I wrote to my family GP pleading for his help. I was delighted when he referred me to a dermatologist who was running trials on this new treatment – and he was looking for volunteers. I agreed.

The drug was called 'Diane'. It was a strong contraceptive pill that worked against the overproduction of testosterone – the hormone that causes acne. It turned out to be the breakthrough that I needed. My confidence and self-esteem started to recover. Every month I was monitored with blood tests and medical checks, but luckily for me, I didn't appear to suffer from any side effects. Gradually, the acne disappeared. The trials were successfully completed, and I remained on Diane for years. I would suffer the odd breakout when I was really upset or stressed, but the lumps cleared much more quickly than before.

Then five years ago, everything changed. My marriage ended and I entered the most painful years of my life. My emotional pain came out in my acne. The medication stopped working overnight. Feeling desperate, I went to see a recommended homeopath in London. Through homeopathic prescriptions of drops and tablets, he gradually brought the problem back under control. The acne started to fade and only broke out when I was really upset.

During these last five years I've also had my biggest life achievements. But, sadly, to accomplish these, I have had to cut off from my parents, former 'friends' and every link with my childhood and marriage. The clearing has been very intense both mentally and physically – in huge outbreaks of acne that even homeopathy couldn't control. It seemed that literally nobody and nothing could help me. I was at my most desperate when my life mentor suggested that I visit Seka.

I attended three healing sessions with Seka over the course of three weeks. The ideal would have been to see her over three consecutive days, but I was very limited by work. But regardless, these visits changed my life.

On the first session Seka told me that my liver was under stress and so I should therefore stop all tablets – both orthodox and homeopathic – immediately. The mere idea of it, let alone the action, absolutely terrified me. How could this possibly work when the problem was so bad even with all the medication? I discussed it with my sister-in-law that evening and she wholeheartedly agreed with Seka. This reassurance gave me the courage to follow Seka's advice. Within days I felt better and the acne faded and left. Seka stressed to me the importance of both a positive attitude and a healthy diet and how these would help to cleanse my system and flush out the toxins.

All was clear for a few months, and then I reached what was to be my last hurdle. I knew in my heart I was clearing my final past issues and, as usual, my skin suffered: the acne flared up to the point where my face was so painful it felt like it was on fire. When this happened, I went to see my GP as soon as I could. As I expected, his recommendations were to restart my old medication and to take an intensive course of antibiotics. My intuition told me to forget the tablets. I went home and was lucky to get an emergency appointment with Seka the following morning.

When I saw her, Seka told me not to worry, because she felt this was the last outbreak. I was to see her once more the following week, by which time, she said, I would be clear. To my absolute amazement, she was right. The lumps were healing by the hour, and the skin between the lumps began to take on a healthy glow. I was speechless. The pain also began to fade until it disappeared completely. When I returned to see Seka six days later, my whole face had almost totally healed. Ten days after the final appointment my skin had completely healed.

I know and appreciate that this is all down to Seka's gift of healing, but as she has explained to me, I also understand that my contribution to this 'team healing effort' is to generate permanent positivity and to look after myself as best I can. Until I met Seka, I didn't believe in miracles. Now I do. Seka has changed my life. The black cloud of low self-esteem and unhappiness has melted away into a new life of freedom and excitement. The problem that darkened most of the years in my life has now left me and, thanks to Seka, I am looking forward to a bright and happy future.

Mariane

Holistic Healing

Over the years, as my English improved, I was able to help my patients on more than a physical level. I had always been able to sense the emotional problems they were facing, but gradually I could speak to them about how to cope with their issues in order to avoid becoming ill again. When I treat someone, my hands read their body. I gather information through my diagnosis by reading their energy as if I'm reading an illustrated poem of their life. It's not something that I consciously do – it's just part and parcel of my gift. I have my own moral code of conduct and that includes doing my job to the best of my ability. It's important to recognize that to heal at the deepest level, we sometimes have to tackle things that seem unrelated, like memories and past situations. I have learned how to raise issues in a gentle and appropriate way, and I find that my patients always feel better afterwards.

One case that really stands out in my mind was when I treated a man who was suffering badly with ME. He was so full of fear that he couldn't sleep at all, but he didn't know where the fear had come from. It was like a black hole, sucking in his energy. He wanted to know where it had started because he realized that he'd never feel truly well until he'd dealt with it. As I was treating him, I started to get some very strong images. I could see that when he was a very young child he had been locked in the garden shed by his father and had been made to stay in there for ten minutes. Although this may seem harmless, the memory of being trapped had coloured his whole life. It was always at the back of his mind, affecting everything he did, so it was no surprise that his body was suffering the consequences. I needed to address this fear and had warned him that things may come up that he couldn't remember. It surprised him that something from many years before that seemed so insignificant was still playing on his mind and affecting his energy. Once we'd cleared this negative memory, his body was open to being totally cured.

Since going to Seka both my physical and my psychic energy have increased enormously. For example, for eight years I had been unable to go to London, firstly due to a knee injury and then due to ME. Since my treatments with Seka I have been to London every week, including a visit to the Tate Gallery and a trip to see the Kirov ballet. I feel that I am quite alive again! My recent visit to Seka had an unexpected beneficial effect too.

I had a very unpleasant childhood, the memories of which were almost totally suppressed until I started psychotherapy five years ago. My feelings of pain, anger and grief were also suppressed. Last week, just as I was settling down to meditate, a friend phoned with some sad and unexpected news and also told me something that made me very angry. I went back to meditate, and within five minutes I could *feel* the anger. I sat there for several minutes aware of the anger, feeling it in a way that I never have before. Several people had told me how to express anger because they were sure that one day I would feel it. So for the first time I was able to get it out of my system, and it felt cathartic. On Thursday a similar thing happened, only this time it was grief over something that had happened two years ago.

Thinking about it, I felt sure that the healing must have enabled me to be aware of these feelings for the first time. I phoned my psychotherapist, who said that he was quite sure that it was: it was a form of healing that I badly needed, and Seka's treatment had brought about this outcome.

Michael

There are times when we need to go back to our past to deal with our memories, but I think that we can often do damage by dwelling on them. It's for this reason that I'm not a great fan of psychotherapy. I've treated many people who've spent years of their life reliving the past, and by going over an event again and again, they never move on. There are certain techniques from the school of neurolinguistic programming which can help you deal with an old emotion in a very short time. If you feel that this would be of use to you, I recommend that you find a qualified NLP practitioner who can help you clear these old memories, and once they've done that, you will be able to focus on your future.

The Lowest Frequency

From my years of healing, I've learned that the most destructive emotion is fear. Fear causes the greatest damage to our health, and it's the cause of so many other negative emotions. If we're lonely, it's often because we are afraid of being alone; if we're worried about work, it's because we're afraid of failing; if we're in an abusive relationship, it may be because we're afraid of walking away; and if we're stuck in an unhappy situation, we are often afraid to change. Fear seeps into every negative emotion, and it has a dense, dark frequency.

As with all other feelings, fear is intangible – we can't see it or touch it. It's not three-dimensional, but we can feel how powerful its energy is. We feel fear in our heart, lungs, skin, hands, feet and our eyes – in fact, I've known people to feel fear almost everywhere in their body. It can be paralysing and it can also be contagious. If we're with someone who is afraid, we can pick up on their fear not only by their verbal or visual signals but also through sensing their fear through their energy, and when there are lots of people together who are afraid, the group energy can be overwhelming.

When I was working in Sarajevo, I had to travel by aeroplane via Rome to Addis Ababa for a work trip. Halfway through the flight I became aware of an unsettled feeling rippling throughout the cabin. The crew informed us that one of the plane's wings was on fire and that we were going to have to make an emergency landing. Everybody started to panic and the energy inside the plane shifted as a result. I could sense the infectious nature of the fear, and the only thing that concerned me was that it would lead to pandemonium. All I could think to do was try to counteract the atmosphere by concentrating on feeling calm, in the hope that my composed vibes might spread around the passengers. The only other person who stayed level-headed was the lady seated next to me: the fear was so powerful that my peace could only impact the person next to me. Luckily, the situation came under control when we landed in Athens. Without this emergency measure, I'm sure the chaos would have taken over.

A great example and one of the best illustrations of the energy of fear was during the attacks on the World Trade Center in New York on 11 September 2001. As the horrific news spread around the globe, the airwaves became dominated by the frequency of terror and everyone tuned into it. We couldn't help it, because the air was so thick with the vibration, and as more people got scared, the frequency became stronger and more overwhelming. Not many people could claim to have been unaffected by this disaster, because it was so powerful, but what few people realized was how much this fear could have affected their health.

When someone is afraid, the worst thing we can do is feel their fear with them. Nervous, jumpy mothers make their children afraid, and that's how phobias are often passed on. A child feels the energy of someone else who is petrified of something – dogs, deep water or spiders – and they learn to be afraid as well. But most fears are irrational and unfounded. The only two innate fears are fear of falling and fear of loud noises, but we have found so many other things to be afraid of. We are afraid of having too little in life and about having too much; of being with other people and of being on our own; we are afraid of death, but we're also scared of all the things that can happen to us whilst we are alive; we are afraid of losing our minds, but it's in our minds that most of our fears are created; we even fear love because if we have someone to love then we're afraid we might lose them. When we look at our fears like this, they seem ridiculous and illogical, and quite often they only become real when we think about them.

The Magic of Laughter

The body can really benefit from some emotions, and one of the best examples of this is laughter. Some people are so convinced of the medicinal properties of laughter that they have set up laughter clubs. These clubs have now been started all over the world, but the idea originated in India in the 1990s. Several years ago I was on holiday in India with a group that was organized by Dr Mosaraf Ali, the celebrity doctor and integrated health expert. I had gone to experience a different culture and also to switch off and take a break. I had been very busy at work, and I wanted to experience a new energy and environment. Dr Ali had arranged for us to attend a laughter club after one of our morning yoga sessions. Our yogi, a toothless old man with the most incredible flexibility, started to lead the laughter. He told us to laugh from our diaphragm and it just seemed so false. There was nothing funny to laugh about! We were just 'ho, ho-ing' and 'ha, ha-ing' and I didn't see the point. I thought he was mad. But after a few minutes of forced laughter people started to giggle naturally, and it soon spread around the group. The frequency of the laughter was so uplifting that we were soon falling about in uncontrollable fits. Having been straight-faced a few moments before, I was in hysterics – and it felt so good!

Research has shown that laughter mitigates the effect of stress hormones in the body, and it also releases growth hormones, which stimulate the immune system.[5] So laughter really does help us to heal ourselves. We also take in a lot more oxygen when we laugh,

5 'Humour Improves Health' *Brain Waves*, Society for Neuroscience, summer 2002.

so we feel invigorated and more awake after a good giggle. It's like taking a natural drug.

I first fell ill in December 2000. I remember that very well because I was celebrating my fortieth birthday and we were returning from Paris on Eurostar. I felt progressively worse as we were nearing the end of our journey, and having made it home, my husband then had to take me straight into casualty. I felt very disconcerted and hazy and was suffering from impaired thinking and tachycardia, which is when your heart rate is too fast. I was admitted to hospital and was wired up to a machine that monitored my heart. For the next week my heart sped up, sometimes reaching 180 beats per minute. This left me exhausted, and the doctors were baffled as to what was causing this. In the end they simply put it down to a virus.

For the next three years I struggled with my health and, to be honest, never regained the level of energy I'd previously had. Several doctors suggested chronic fatigue syndrome, or ME, and I seemed to fit the bill as I had all the symptoms. In March 2004 I had a relapse and couldn't move from my bed. I felt so ill I wasn't able to eat and just walking to the bathroom would leave me breathless and exhausted. My heart rate started to speed up again. My husband and I were getting to the end of our tether with my mysterious illness, and we said we'd pay to see as many private doctors as we could to sort out this problem once and for all.

First we saw an endocrinologist who gave me the all clear, but suspected I had a heart problem, so he referred me to his colleague at the Brompton Hospital. The cardiologist was sure I had SVT, which is an electrical fault with the heart, and wanted to do ablation therapy. I was unhappy with this diagnosis as I was with the doctor for less than ten minutes. He ignored my other symptoms (which he called 'all the other stuff') and seemed happy to go ahead with the procedure without doing any tests on me. I would have had to have a pacemaker for the rest of my life and that seemed crazy.

My husband was very frustrated by this time. He is a Cambridge-educated engineer so he's quite a logical person by nature, and he couldn't understand the doctors' approaches to diagnosis. We didn't know where to turn next.

My neighbour told me about her friend's daughter who had been to a healer called Seka Nikolic. She had helped her after she'd been bedridden for nine years, so my husband and I figured we had nothing to lose. I didn't know anything about healers or healing, and my husband, being a scientist, was very sceptical, but he said he'd take me. We booked seven appointments with Seka at the Hale Clinic, and I can remember thinking, 'How am I going to make the journey into London? How will I walk from the car to the clinic?'

I was so exhausted as I sat in reception that I remember half-lying and half-sitting, propping myself up on cushions and feeling desperate to be back in my bed! I recall Seka calling me in to the room, and I was surprised by her appearance. I know it seems stupid, but I'd imagined a healer to look like a hippy or a gypsy with lots of bangles and long, black hair. Seka was the complete opposite: she was a very attractive blonde in a pinstripe suit and she looked like a business-woman. This was my first surprise.

I told Seka my history, and she told me to lie down on the couch. She placed her hands on my head, then on my throat and then over my left ear. Her hand immediately felt very warm, and my ear got quite hot. 'Here is where the trouble is,' she announced. I was amazed as I'd been telling everyone I'd had ear pain after I'd suffered from a dreadful sore throat but I hadn't mentioned it to Seka. Somehow she picked up on it anyway. She then put her hands on my chest, and I can only describe what felt like butterflies moving. One of my symptoms is a tingling sensation in my body, which Seka said she could also feel but she didn't think there was anything wrong with my heart. She said this with such easy, relaxed confidence, and I found myself believing her.

After the treatments my husband and I slowly made our way back to the car. My husband asked me how I felt, and we will both never forget that day because as he asked me the strangest thing happened. I started to laugh and laugh, and laugh and pretty soon I was in uncontrollable fits of laughter. Tears were streaming down my face. My husband joined in and hugged me. He said, 'Chris, I never thought I'd hear you like that again.' We must have looked a strange sight, laughing and hugging and crying.

The second unexpected thing happened as soon as I got home. For the first time in months I felt absolutely starving. I had lost a lot of weight and was reacting to almost everything I tried to eat. But now I felt a strong desire for a curry! My husband got a takeaway, and I ate until I thought I would burst. That meal tasted so good, and my husband and my mum, who'd come over, were looking at each other in amazement. Just seeing their faces made me laugh. They had been trying to get me to eat for ages, and here I was, after just one treatment with Seka, scoffing food down like a pig. I then slept for the rest of the day.

The next day I told Seka about the laughing. She explained that this was the energy block releasing and she wasn't the least bit surprised. 'That's good,' she said. 'Most people cry, but I think it's better to laugh!'

After another treatment I had the worst headache ever, and again, Seka said this was the releasing of energy. She said that my body was in a state of exhaustion but that she knew I'd get better. I remember being surprised when she suggested I do some exercise, like cycling or going for a walk. I was hardly able to walk upstairs without collapsing. But I persevered, and one day a friend came over to prop me up on her side while we walked around the block.

I was improving slowly, and a couple of weeks later I had another block of treatments. This block seemed to really give me a boost, and I have no doubt that Seka kick-started the process of my body getting better. I've continued to improve and now see Seka on a maintenance basis. I still don't know how she works, but I have no doubt that she has helped me and continues to do so. I just hope she never retires!

Seka has now treated my sceptical husband too. When he saw my results, he thought he'd see her for an ongoing back problem, which he'd had for years. His back has been considerably better, and he even managed to carry our eight-year-old daughter home from our friends' house after she'd fallen asleep. There's no way he would have been able to do that before.

Chris Gale

So you see, you don't have to go to a laughter club to experience this healing power, and you don't have to wait until something makes you laugh. Children find a lot to laugh about in the day, but when we grow up, we become a lot more serious and so we can sometimes go through the whole day with only a few light moments. So why not have a spontaneous laugh any time? It's best if you find at least one other person to do this with and then you just force yourself to laugh. I know it sounds ridiculous – and that's what I thought at first – but believe me, once you feel how great it is, you'll wish you'd done it sooner. I've known people to regret wallowing in negative emotions, but I've never known anybody regret having a good laugh.

9

DEALING WITH STRESS

During my years of healing I've noticed patterns as to why people become ill. There's no doubt that illness sometimes comes about because of accidents, infection or the environment; however, what I'm seeing more and more as our world continues to develop is that illness grows out of people's unhappiness. There are many things that make up a happy life, and these things all play a role in determining our health, so it seems to me that a lot of disease is caused by a lack of ease, or 'dis-ease', with our lives. I don't have the answers to all the world's problems, but I do know that the way in which we choose to live has significant repercussions on how we feel. The good news is that everybody can learn how to be aware of how their choices in life affect their energy shifts so that they can manage their health.

Great Expectations

As society moves more quickly, so do our expectations. Time and time again I see people put themselves under pressure to strive for things that they feel they 'should' have. We think more about what we want than what we need, falling into the temptation of wanting what others have, desiring what we think would make us happy and lusting after the things we see other people have. As we focus on material things, it becomes easy to lose touch with who we are, why we're here and what we really need to make us happy and healthy.

When I was working in Sarajevo, I was sent on a business trip to Ethiopia. I was so lucky to be able to travel around and see some of the country, and I was taken to some remote areas. The Ethiopians were so generous, wanting to give me presents at every opportunity. They had so little, but they thought nothing of giving it away. I helped to make coffee, which took nearly three hours to prepare. We picked, cleaned and ground the beans by hand – a far cry from the cappuccino that I was used to being served but my hosts thought nothing of it. The village I stayed in had an atmosphere of celebration, as if every day were a festival. These people had one of the simplest lifestyles on the planet and had very little in the way of material wealth. My life changed during this trip because it was the first time I had seen people be so joyous about the little things in life. I started to ask myself what was really important in life: what do we really need, and what do we simply want? I realized that happiness doesn't come from having things but from a balanced state of being, and I felt honoured to have spent time with people who had such strong spirit and energy.

Living a simple life doesn't have to mean going without. I believe that when people find a balance between what they need and what they want, they reach a point where they experience a smooth flow of energy and they vibrate powerfully at a healthy frequency.

The Stress Epidemic

Stress is a word that we use all too often. It never used to exist, yet nowadays it's used frequently and generously. It used to describe situations that were extreme, but it's become a catch-all word to explain all sorts of inconvenience and mishap: 'I've just had the most stressful bus ride', 'He didn't call me back – I'm stressed out', 'The children are stressed about their maths test' and 'I'm so stressed – I've put on two pounds!' You may have laughed at these examples, but they're all things that I've heard people say. It's normal for humans to experience moderate amounts of stress; in fact, we need a certain amount of stress to get out of bed in the morning. But stress levels now far exceed this natural, manageable level. The pressures of life are growing and so is the speed at which the world moves, but what many of us are failing to do is learn how to cope with these changes.

I believe that stress is often an excuse for failure – a reaction to the realization that we can't cope. Being stressed at work often masks our anger that we're in over our head; getting stressed out in a traffic jam is usually because of our inability to relax; and stress in relationships is sometimes a sign that we need to get out. If we're stressed by something that we have the power to change, then we should do it. This may sound harsh, but if we just look at the hard facts we remove a lot of the emotion that can keep us stuck in an uncomfortable place. If our stress is caused by an inability to cope, we either need to learn to deal with the situation or remove ourselves from it.

But what about if our stress is because of something we can't change? What do we do then? If you live in a remote part of the countryside and you get snowed in, what's the point in getting wound up? The whole point of living in the country is to get away from built-up areas, so there's a risk that you may get cut off. You chose to live there, so you can either learn to live with it or you can move. If you live in a major city and you get stuck in traffic, don't tell me you're surprised! You have to accept the traffic as part and parcel of your life choice, so adapt to fit it. People who don't get stressed are often those who realize the difference between things they can do something about and things that are beyond their control. They see that they have a choice of what they do and how they feel, and it's very empowering. Once you see how much stress plays a role in creating illness, you may choose to think like that as well.

When I first came to London, I had no idea what stress was. When patients used to say, 'I'm stressed,' I couldn't understand what they meant, and the phrase didn't translate well into Serbo-Croat! The only other place where I had spent a lot of time was in Lanzarote and that wasn't a stressful place either. Gradually, I started to understand what stress was. As my patients explained what was causing their stress, I realized that what they were talking about was life itself. There always have been and there always will be things that challenge us, and that's how we thrive and grow. But when we feel that we can't deal with the challenge, that's when stress becomes an issue.

When we experience a stressful situation, our physiology changes. Our body becomes flooded with stress hormones like adrenalin and cortisol, and these chemicals induce what is known as the 'fight or flight response'. Whilst we are rarely exposed to real physical threats as we used to be, our bodies have yet to evolve to recognize this and we still react as if we're about to be attacked. As we prepare to run away or fight, our heart races, our breathing becomes rapid and shallow and our blood flow is diverted from normal metabolic activities to feed our muscles – and one of the systems that suffers the most is our immune system. So it's straightforward really: being stressed can disrupt our energy to the point where we become vulnerable to illness.

Let's take a moment to think about the frequency of stress. I would guess that most of you have been in a situation in which you've been stressed by transport – say you've been in a traffic jam or on a bus or a train that was delayed. You can probably think back to where you were and recall the feeling: there were lots of people sitting around feeling the same negative emotion, wondering, 'When are we going to get out of this?' One by one people started to fidget and tut. They looked at their watches and shook their heads. Maybe some even started to get really frustrated and clenched their fists. You just knew that pulses were racing, blood pressure was rising, and the level of dis-ease was growing. This is stress en masse – and it's incredibly powerful in its negativity. The frequency of the energy is low, and it starts to take its toll on your body – unless you learn to let it go.

Stress is damaging. It leaves us tired and weak, and when we're exhausted, we find it harder to notice how our body is feeling, and this is when we can fail to see the signs of illness. Our energy is vibrating uncomfortably, and sometimes we simply don't notice.

I had been suffering from a terrible aching neck and stomach problems for about six months when I first went to see Seka. She was recommended to me by a friend, and I decided that I had nothing to lose by going to see her. I had no idea what was wrong with me, as my GP could find nothing wrong, but I was convinced that I had some kind of illness.

Seka didn't ask me anything about myself and simply started treating me. She began by placing her hands at the base of my skull. Almost immediately the pain and tightness in my neck, which I'd become so used to, disappeared. I assumed this must be because I was lying down and didn't think anything more about it. I just lay there very still, – not knowing what to expect. After about five minutes, by which time I was feeling incredibly relaxed, Seka placed her hands on my head and said to me, 'This is where your problems are. You are always stressed about things.' I thought this was a general comment and was still waiting for her to tell me what was wrong. As she moved down to my stomach area, I could feel the most wonderful glowing sensation in the whole abdominal area and was beginning to feel as if I was floating. I didn't want to get up when the treatment was finished!

At the end of the session I asked Seka what was wrong with me and she said, 'It is all stress. You are grinding your teeth in your sleep and that is causing your neck pain. Your stomach is also reacting badly – all because of stress.'

I was surprised that this was all Seka had found, and I was also very embarrassed that the discomfort and distress I'd been feeling was because of my own behaviour. It would have been so much easier to deal with if it had been due to some kind of illness because then I wouldn't have to face the fact that I needed to change the way I was living if I wanted my health to improve.

Seka continued to treat me for the rest of the week, during which time my neck totally eased up and my stomach pains eased. She gave me advice on how to manage my stress so that I could keep myself in that healthy state. I started to reduce my work hours and also took up meditation, which was something I had been toying with for a while, but I never thought I had enough time! I can see now, though, how important these changes have been to my health.

Seka made me realize that we have to do everything in our power to take care of our health and since then I haven't allowed myself to get in such a state again.

Jane

Increase Your Own Awareness

If you're serious about improving your health, you have to become aware of what your energy is doing. We often only notice that something's wrong when we're really unwell, but it's much more effective to pick up on the early signs. Our bodies are constantly giving us feedback, and everyone experiences different symptoms. Some of the most common signals that your energy is off balance are:

- Headaches

- Backache

- Disturbed sleep

- Significant change in appetite

- Unusual tiredness

- Lack of concentration

- Aching limbs

- Knotty stomach

Our energy is personal, but these signs are pretty universal, and you will have particular symptoms that you're more likely to experience. You may look at this list and think, 'That's normal, isn't it? I'm not ill if I feel like that.' And you'd be right. You're not ill – yet – but your body is giving you the warning signs that if you don't correct your frequency when it's just starting to wobble, you risk crashing.

Getting rid of symptoms is one thing, but if you're serious about managing your health in the long run, the next step is to find the cause of your stress. One of the best ways to do this is to imagine that someone has been filming you on a hidden camera and they give you the tape. In your mind, rewind the tape back to a point where you feel you began to feel stressed and play back the film as if you're watching it on a large cinema screen. Be conscious of staying detached from what's going on, as if you're an observer. By stepping back from our lives, we can see what our weaknesses and issues are, and once we've discovered them, we can start to deal with them to avoid bouts of stress in the future.

I believe that we all have an intuitive sense of what we should be doing with our lives and what's best for us, but few of us pay any attention to it. Our energy is like our navigation system – when we're on the right track, our energy vibrates strongly, but when we veer off, it drops, and that's the time to do something about it. As I have found through healing people, the more we ignore our instincts, the further we get from our natural frequency – or to put it another way, the more we feel a dis-ease with life, the more we open ourselves to the possibility of sickness. We are all susceptible to changes in energy, and even fame and wealth can't buy us health and happiness.

The Pressure of the Limelight

'Hectic schedules and jet-setting around the globe can wreak havoc with even the most seasoned fashion insider's energy levels.' This was the opening to a recent newspaper article about me.[1] The piece was about how A-listers maintain their health when they have so many social and work commitments, and they called me 'the Energy Giver'. It's true that I have treated many celebrities, something that the press has loved to report on, but I'm not like a fashion accessory to them: they come for genuine reasons. Those of us who don't have a celebrity lifestyle find it hard to imagine what it's like to be faced with constant media demands and to be continually worried about being caught on camera. Rather than coming with a specific ailment, many celebrities visit me for an energy boost so that they can cope with their hectic lives. Whether they sing, act or compete, the amount of energy they exude when they're performing can leave them drained and down. By giving so much of themselves, they can lose touch with their natural frequency and the balance that they need to maintain their health.

1 Maria McErlane, 'A Time to Heal', *Sunday Times Style Magazine*, 19 September, 2004.

I've had two lots of treatment with Seka, but I admit that it wasn't my idea to see her! I was coming up to an important competition and was pushing myself hard – as usual. A very good friend recommended that I see Seka. He said that he'd been seeing her for years and that she'd really be able to re-energize me. I was sceptical about going. I had never had any kind of alternative treatment before, and I was a bit cynical about how effective she could be. I had no idea what to expect, but it was all straightforward. I found the treatments really relaxing, and it was just a novelty to lie down still for half an hour.

Immediately after the first session I could feel a difference. It's funny for me to hear myself say that after being so cynical, but I really could feel the change in my energy. I continued to see Seka for the whole week, and each day I got more of a buzz. By the end of the sessions I had so much more energy than when I'd started out – and not just physically. I was mentally more alert and found it easier to focus on my game. I was generally feeling healthier, and it was as if life had come back to me.

Ronnie O'Sullivan, former snooker World Champion

To me, fame seems like a strange concept. I can't imagine what it's like to have your life so much in the public eye. It seems that just because you're well known or you have a special talent that you can't have your privacy. Many celebrities find that when their performance or competition is over, they want to revert back to having a private existence, but the media and the public always expect them to be on form, demanding a piece of them at every opportunity.

I treat many celebrities and athletes before and after they perform, to help them keep up their energy levels and stay balanced. I suppose the closest I've got to experiencing demands like this was when I first discovered my gift back in Sarajevo. People used to mob me in the street and follow me home, and I hated it. I didn't feel safe, and I had to get away from the attention. Nowadays I cherish the fact that I can walk down the street and be anonymous and that I can go out for dinner with nobody watching me. They're only simple things, but they make all the difference to me.

One of my regular patients and close friends is Lolicia Aitken. After facing a scandalous time with her ex-husband, she left the UK to get away from the strain of the situation. I visited her in Switzerland every few weeks to treat her and help her regain her energy: prolonged stress had left her vibrating at a very low frequency. Her nightmares stopped almost immediately after I started treating her, and her case was reported in the *Daily Mail*. She told the paper, 'I could have ended up as a shallow socialite with a drink problem. That's why so many rich people are unhappy, because they don't know where to go, they have no direction. When you have everything, do you turn to drink, drugs or destruction?' The pressure of public life had left Lolicia confused and drained. By learning to recognize and balance her energy, she has learned to live in the present and to deal with whatever is thrown at her.

Sometimes we move so fast that we don't notice what's going on inside our body. And sometimes we know something's wrong and we don't want to face up to it – it's called denial. If a child tells you that they don't feel well, you don't ignore them and tell them to carry on; you listen to what they have to say. For many people, it's time to listen to the messages that their own body is giving them and face up to what's wrong.

Making a Living Can Ruin Your Life

Most of us have to work at some point in our lives, and some people see work simply as something they have to do to be able to enjoy the rest of their life. But we spend a significant proportion of time in the workplace, and even when we're 'out of hours', many of us still think about our jobs, so it's only natural for our work to impact on our happiness and our health. How many people do you know who genuinely love what they do? How many people look forward to going to work because they're proud of what they achieve? I know lots of people who dislike their jobs, and given that we spend most of our waking hours at work, a dreary job can be a major cause of stress. I've found that most of my patients aren't in the most suitable jobs for them, and a lot of the time their body's telling them it's not right – they just don't read the signs.

I treated one man who had a very powerful artistic energy. I sensed this as soon as I started treating him and wasn't at all surprised when he talked about how his desk job was running him into the ground. His attitude was affecting his health as he had allowed himself to become out of tune with his talents and his natural vibration. After his treatments he gave up his job and is now a successful – and healthy – artist.

Our work is an expression of who we are. I had studied hard for many years to get my job in marketing, and whilst I enjoyed it and could do it well, there was obviously something else that I had to do! My story is a bit different in that my job found me, as opposed to me discovering it, but nevertheless we are all given signs as to what we are gifted to do – it's whether we choose to follow them.

Does Money Make the World Go Round?

One of the main things that affects our decision to work is money. We need enough money to satisfy our key needs – like food, clothing and shelter – but some of us 'need' money to satisfy all our other wants. Everyone has their own interpretation of what money can bring, and after I came to live in the UK, where everything was much more expensive than I was used to, I underwent a big shift in the way I viewed the value of money.

It wasn't long after I'd moved to London that I travelled to the Middle East to treat one of my patients who was too ill to come to me. When I was due to return home, this lady offered me a very significant amount of money to stay for one more week. This offer put me at a crossroads: having just moved to the UK, I could really have done with the money to help me buy a house and it would have relieved me of a huge burden. But I also knew that I had done everything I could for her. The extra week may have made a slight difference to her recovery, but not enough for me to justify such a generous amount of money. My conscience told me that it would be wrong to take this money, and I knew that by taking up the offer I'd be cheating my patient. I wasn't prepared to do that. I wouldn't have been able to sleep at night.

Money is a very powerful force, and we can act very differently when we're tempted by it. It's important to remain in control of money rather than letting it control us. From what I've learned, you can make money your prime concern but it won't buy you contentment. I've treated people who have more money than you could imagine, but they still experience drops in energy and illness – and they're not always happy. If you follow your heart and focus on enjoying what you do, money will come to you. It can be frightening sometimes to trust yourself, but it's rare to find a person whose happiness and health come solely from their bank balance.

Do You Want to Break Free?

There are many ways that we can trap ourselves in an uncomfortable place. You may be aware that you're stuck in a rut but have no idea how to get out, so let's see what may be keeping you there.

Imagine someone has been in a job that they hate for ten years.

They fell into it by accident, and they've found themselves putting up with it even though they know deep down that it isn't satisfying them. What keeps them there? Why do they spend so much time feeling heavy inside? Let's take another example. I'm sure you all know someone who has been in a damaging relationship, yet they stayed in it way after they knew it was wrong. They put up with a mediocre life when they knew they deserved better. Why would anyone do that? Why would anyone put up with second or even third best? The answer is habit.

We are creatures of habit. We do many of the same things in the same way over and over again. We wake up, wash and get dressed; we brush our teeth automatically; we drive our cars without thinking about what we're doing; we check our emails and type automatically; we often eat the same things at the same times of day; we watch the same programmes on television; we go to the same coffee shops; and we say the same things repeatedly. We have routines that we follow day in and day out – and this ability to follow patterns of thought and behaviour means that we are very efficient! Our habits help us to get through each day without having to relearn everything from scratch. But as well as these useful habits, we all have some automatic thoughts and emotions that aren't helpful to us at all.

One example of this that I often see is the habit that many people fall into when they're ill. They get used to being weak, and they accept the fact that their life is limited by their illness, and even when they're healed, they still fear becoming ill again. They have become so used to being a victim of their disease that they can't remember how to be free and healthy.

I remember treating one lady, Nicola O'Ferrall. Prior to contracting ME, Nicola had been very energetic and had been a keen marathon runner. She had a very good relationship with her GP and so she found herself very sceptical of my treatments. Nevertheless, she came to me on recommendation and noticed a huge difference after the first treatment. During the week I suggested that Nicola went for a swim. She seemed surprised. She was accustomed to being inactive even though she used to love exercising. She had been ill for so long that she couldn't remember what it felt like to use her energy. She told the *Guardian* newspaper, 'After three days I swam twenty lengths. I was so suspicious that I took the water they gave me before each treatment for analysis. I'm now fine, fingers crossed.' Needless to say, Nicola needn't have been afraid of the water – it was free of any suspicious substances! The thing she should have been wary of was her own brain, which wanted to keep her within her comfort zone of being ill.

Our brains are like computers, and our habits are like computer programs. Once we programme a habit into our brain, it runs automatically – until we change the programme. Since I have been in the UK I have come to learn a lot about re-programming our minds. Through my friendship with Paul McKenna I learned about neurolinguistic programming (NLP). NLP is a scientific method of looking at the ways in which we programme our behaviour and thought patterns, and I have found it to be one of the most valuable tools in helping people relearn how to be healthy. Helping clients have a change of attitude is the hardest part of my work. My healing comes naturally to me – it's something I do out of habit – and if I tried to think about it, I probably couldn't do it! But I always need to think carefully about how I help someone to change their thoughts.

I find it most effective if I give people suggestions and challenges right from the start of their treatment. I know how quickly someone's body can change. It's important, therefore, that the mind is ready to deal with the change so that my work isn't undone. I also like to give people just a few key messages to prevent them from getting confused, and on the first day I set out goals for what I think they will achieve by the end of the week. I often get a shocked or negative response from patients at this stage because they think I'm crazy! They think I don't understand how they feel and that my suggestions are ridiculous. But the opposite is true. I have treated so many people that I can tell very early on how well someone will adapt and how quickly they'll accept their healing. And I can also spot the people who like having problems – people who are so used to being the victim that they've forgotten how to be strong.

One lady came to me because she couldn't stop sneezing. She would sneeze every few minutes, and her sneezes were really violent. She'd been to see many doctors, and none of them had come up with any cures, they had just given her a monitor that measured the power of her sneeze. Her husband, who came with her, would rush over to her every time she sneezed to take the measurement. He was following her around like a puppy and pandering to her condition. During the first treatment I could see that what she really needed to do was sneeze away her husband: the more he ran around after her, the more she sneezed. She had no incentive to get rid of her sneezing because it got her attention and care. Their lives had been so dominated by this problem that when it went away, I wondered what either of them would do with themselves.

It's always easier to help someone else because we can stand back from their situation and see the best path for them. When we try to change our own behaviour, it's much harder, because we're so embroiled in our own lives. Some of the toughest cases I've had have been psychotherapists, coaches and counsellors: they work at helping other people change their patterns, but they usually find it really hard to do the same themselves.

Being Positive Is a Choice

Whilst my job is first and foremost to treat my clients with Bio-Energy, I have found that helping them change the way they react to negative situations is vital in avoiding potential relapses. I'm sure you can see by now that many illnesses come about because of emotional blocks, and by showing people how to deal with these, I'm helping them achieve the best state of health possible. But I know that once my patients leave the clinic they're on their own, so I have to make the best use of the time I get with them to show them that they always have a choice.

I'm sure you've heard this before, but it really is helpful to be able to see the good in everything. If we go through life always seeing the bad and the ugly, we'll continue to damage our energy and will find it hard to heal ourselves. Any woman who's had a baby will tell you that childbirth is painful, but they'll also tell you that the joy of having a baby far outweighs the agony. There was a time when I was unable to drive for a while. I was so used to driving that it seemed impossible to be without a car. But I knew I couldn't change the situation so all I could do was change my reaction to it. Because I find public transport very draining, I started to walk everywhere. I saw London in a whole new light and discovered parts of the city I had never seen before. I walked through Regent's Park every day to get between clinics and I grew to love that open space. I also got fitter and lost weight – so there were lots of benefits!

One of the hardest times in my life was when my country was at war. I had grown up mixing with people from all cultures and religions. I went to school with Muslims, Serbs and Croats – I just saw them as people and that was how I knew my country to be. When war broke out, I saw neighbours fighting with neighbours and brothers fighting with brothers. It went against all the beliefs I had grown up with, and as far as I could see, they were forced to kill each other by the political situation. It was a challenge to be positive. I helped my family to move to safety, and I made sure they had what they needed. As my home got destroyed, I found myself without roots and so I made the best of what I had. I was in Lanzarote during the war, and even though I wasn't there for a long time, I still made a home for myself. I couldn't make the war stop, but I could do my best for my family, friends and for me. If I had given in to the war and let its frequency disturb my energy, I'm in no doubt that I would have become ill.

The Answer Lies Within Us

Every single element of our life affects our energy: the work we do, the people we spend time with, our lifestyle and the way we think. All of these choices have an impact on the vibration of our energy, which means that they all also affect our health. If we lose touch with what we need to be fulfilled and nourished, then the things that should be life's pleasures often become life's enemies. When we do a job that doesn't use our natural strengths, or we spend time with someone whose ethics are very different to ours, we feel dis-ease inside us. It may be a churning stomach, a knot in our heart, energy crashes, persistent headaches or a stiff back. Often our energy is telling us through these physical signs that it's not right – our frequency is off track and our body wants us to pay attention.

I remember when I was in a relationship that wasn't right for me. I tried to make it right – I desperately wanted the other person to fit what I wanted and needed, but ultimately it was wrong. If you have to force someone to be very different to who they naturally are, then it will damage both your energy and theirs, just as trying to be something you're not will affect you. But when you find or do something that's right for you, it just feels good. Leaving Sarajevo was the right thing for me, and whilst I could have found lots of reasons to stay – my family, my friends and the fact I didn't speak English – I still left. I didn't analyse my decision; I followed my energy and my intuition.

We need to learn to be aware of our energy and how it is affected by our choices. If we allow ourselves to feel discontented or ill at ease, we leave ourselves vulnerable to illness. A key step in self-healing is being in touch with our natural vibration. If we can tell when our energy is shifting, we can correct it, but if we let our stresses take root and grow, our dis-ease can become a precursor to more serious illnesses. We are the only people who really know how we feel inside, so we need to take responsibility for our health and have the courage to follow our instinct.

10

A PROGRAMME FOR SELF-HEALING

One question that I often get asked is 'How do you heal yourself?' The answer is that I maintain my health through being very aware of my body. What I aim to do for all of my patients is teach them to maintain their own health in the same way. It's the only sensible option for the long term – after all, who wants to rely on other people forever? For most people, I suggest that they leave longer periods of time between booster treatments with me and that they start to realize the importance of their own lifestyle choices.

By the time you get to this final chapter your mind will probably be buzzing with new ideas and experiences, so I want to highlight what I see as the most important ideas in order for you to be able to work on your own energy. I hope you will have learned about yourself through reading about my experiences and those of my patients, but the best way to do this is to turn your attention inside. In this section I have pulled together all of the tips and suggestions that I use with my patients so that you have an easy-to-follow programme to help you heal yourself. Some of the information has already been said in other parts of the book, but by including it here, you will be able to refer back to this section time and time again and find everything you need.

What is Self-healing?

A lot of people try Bio-Energy healing when all else has failed and they can't help themselves. My patients have often been suffering for months, even years, before they come to see me. Every time I treat someone who is seriously ill it reiterates my fundamental belief that we shouldn't wait until we're really sick to pay attention to our health. I have confidence that each and every one of us is able to become aware of the subtle changes in our energy, which if left unchecked, lead to more serious things. We can all heal ourselves on a daily basis. It's what many people would call preventative medicine, but in my eyes, it's the simplest form of healing – and it's all about being self-aware and keeping a balanced state of mind and body.

As you now know, healing takes place in the mind as well as in the body. Whether someone is suffering from a physical or emotional disease, they always need to look at how they think. Some people seem to keep themselves in good health, whilst others find that they're often ill. Although our reactions to illness are affected by what the illness is and how serious it is, it seems that there are other clues within our personality as to how we are likely to react to being unwell. Research has shown that a depressed mental state has a direct negative impact on the immune system, not only causing illness but also extending the recovery time. I'm sure I'm not alone in my belief that pessimism attracts poor health and negativity, and that happy and positive feelings attract vitality and robust health.

Dr Bernard Grad, of McGill University in Montreal, undertook a series of experiments looking at the effects of positive and negative energy on the growth of plants.[1] He used healers to give

1 Dr Bernard Grad (ed. G. Schmeidler), 'The Biological Effects of the "Laying-on-of-Hands" on Animals and Plants: Implications for Biology', *Parapsychology: Its Relation to Physics, Biology and Psychiatry* (New Jersey, 1967).

positive energy and selected people suffering from depression for the negative. Grad took barley seeds and made them 'unwell' by soaking them in salty water, which is known to stunt the growth of plants. Rather than working directly on the plant, the healers and depressed people energized the containers of salt water without using physical contact with the water. The seeds were then placed either in pots of the healer-treated salt water or salt water treated by the unhappy people, or in a third pot containing untreated salt water. The plants that grew in the healer-treated water were taller and had a higher chlorophyll content than those in the control group, and those that were planted in the salt water that was energized by the depressives, when compared to the control group, were stunted in their growth.

Grad also showed that you don't have to be a professional healer to have a positive effect on health. He repeated the experiment using a group of 'green-thumbed' gardeners. He found that they managed to nurture the water in a similar way to the healers and achieved the same increased growth rate in the plants. This shows that everyone has an ability to heal and that this ability is affected by our mental state. But whilst research can play an important role in proving this, I have seen through my own healing experiences that one of the strongest predictors of health is someone's emotional state.

How Do We Self-heal?

In my experience everything we do, say and feel affects our health, so to live a balanced life we need to keep our emotions stable and happy. When our emotions nourish us, our energy is strong, and when our energy is strong, our health is good. By living the life that is meant for us, we heal ourselves at a fundamental level. This may seem like a sweeping statement so I have broken this down into ten simple things that you can follow as a self-healing programme: listen to your intuition; nurture your creativity; keep active; eat energy-giving foods; practise energy breathing; know your limitations; protect yourself from negative energy; avoid electromagnetic pollution and geopathic stress; manage your emotions; and keep growing.

1. Be Intuitive

We all have a sixth sense – an intuition that tells us when we're feeling happy with life or when something isn't right. We're born with this instinct, but sadly, many of us have lost touch with it. When we talk about being 'out of sorts', 'off colour', 'under the weather' or 'out of kilter', we're describing the feeling we get when our natural frequency is out of tune. We usually feel like this because we don't feel balanced, grounded or rooted in a healthy state. Our imbalance can be physical – for example, we could be coming down with a cold, our hormones could be out of balance or we could simply be worn out. Or our imbalance can be a sign that we are emotionally out of kilter. This kind of shift in energy can be caused by things like unresolved anger after an argument, anxiety over an upcoming event or a general frustration with life.

Some neuroscientists have researched how and why we can feel this sixth sense at work in our body. It seems that our intestines are lined with masses of nerve cells, so it seems entirely possible that the density of receptors in the intestines may be why we feel many emotions in that part of the body.[2] So whilst we may not always be consciously aware of our intuitive sense, we can feel it in our intestines – hence the term 'gut instinct'.

All the major decisions that I've taken in my life have been

2 Candace Pert, Ph.D, *Molecules of Emotion: Why You Feel the Way You Do* (London, 1997).

based on my gut feeling. I left Yugoslavia to move to the Canary Islands, and then I moved from the Canaries to the UK, and on both these occasions I left within days of deciding. I just knew that what I was doing was right for me. I've always followed my survival instinct, and I was taught from a young age to trust in my feelings. I've come to learn not to analyse a situation. When you question something, you will always find a reason not to do it: why it's not sensible, why it's not the right time, or why it's safer to stay as you are. But when you make a decision without questioning, you know that your intuition is guiding you and it must be right. You have to recognize this and trust yourself, and in my experience if you do this, things always work out. But to be able to listen to our intuition and do the right thing, we have to be aware of what's going on around us and inside us.

One thing that I've learned from treating and observing people is that we can be physically in the present moment whilst being emotionally stuck in the past or the future. Don't get me wrong – I think it's important to know where your future is headed, but once you've set yourself on the right path, the only way to get there is by focusing on the here and now. Whatever you do in the next minute, hour and day will play a part in creating your future. I learned that when I moved to the UK. I sensed that London would be my home for a long time, but if I looked too far ahead, beyond a time when I felt safe and comfortable, I'd get afraid. Everything was so new and strange to me that all I could do was to trust my own actions, each day, to help me build my future.

We can rationalize a situation until we're blue in the face, but deep down we know what's best for us – we just feel it. Each and every one of us has an instinct, which tells us when something sits well with us or when it doesn't, and following our instinct is essential for self-healing. It may sound obvious, but when we make the right intuitive choices, we feel good – we literally buzz or vibrate at the right level – and when our body and mind are in balance, our intuition opens up. When we make a poor choice, we feel it too. It may be a sinking feeling or a lump in our stomach; perhaps we can't sleep at night, or we have no appetite; or maybe we have a recurring injury or physical condition. By moving from our natural frequency, we leave ourselves open to niggles and dis-ease, and I really believe that when we're in an unhealthy state, we make unhealthy decisions.

Think back to a time when you didn't listen to your gut instinct, a time when you sensed that you should make one choice, but you did something else. What happened as a result? Often in these cases, we end up missing a train, taking the wrong job or getting stuck in a draining relationship. Looking back to situations like these, we can see that we knew deep down that our choice was wrong, but we went with it anyway.

When we find something we really need in our life, there is no struggle. When we meet the right partner or friend, things just seem to come together, even against the odds. If the perfect job comes along, it feels right and we find ourselves not wanting to question it. And when we walk into our future home, our energy starts to feel positive and strong. It can be scary to go with the flow of our intuition but, chances are, it's the best thing for us.

If we are unwell, our intuition usually tries to tell us how to cure ourselves. We get messages from our body about what to do and what to stop doing. Perhaps we get a sign that we need to rest, a heavy, sick feeling after eating certain foods, or an uneasy feeling every time we're with a particular person. When I was in hospital with my gallstones, despite the doctors' recommendations that I have an operation to remove them, I knew that it wasn't the right thing. I found out a while after that the doctor who would have operated on me was mentally unstable and had been malpractising. If you remember, it was during this illness that I had the urge to eat food that was totally wrong for me. The last thing I should have been eating was heavy pastries, but I knew as soon as I saw and smelt them that they were what I needed, and they worked like a magic pill. I wouldn't necessarily recommend this, as it could have been very dangerous, but for some reason, after a meagre drip-feed of chamomile, the shock of the solid food kick-started my body. I just happened to be lucky that my instincts had been right and this was a very particular situation.

Similarly, pregnant women often crave the strangest things because their body lacks certain nutrients; for example, when you hear rare cases of women craving coal and unusual foodstuffs. And children sometimes eat odd things, like plaster from walls or ants, because they need some of the nutrients. These are great examples of listening to your intuition.

The most important way to heal ourselves is to make the right choices in life: in our job, our relationships and our lifestyle. Someone may follow in their father's footsteps because that's what's expected of them, but if that profession isn't right for them, they'll suffer for the rest of their life. Similarly, if we get stuck in an unhappy relationship, say for the sake of our children, we will eventually feel the effect of this in our health. We know what to do – we just have to trust in ourselves. Intuition is like a muscle: if we don't use it, it becomes weak, but when we exercise it consistently it grows stronger and more powerful.

If we are heading on the right path, our body will send us signs that our energy has shifted, but it can be all too easy to miss these warning signs. We usually only pick up on them when the signs are obvious and we're really unwell. It's much easier to correct our energy frequency when it's just started to shift, and when we pay attention to what's happening to our energy on a daily basis, this becomes second nature. After a while you will be able to tune in to your own vibrations and pick up on your body's particular symptoms without having to think about it.

Whilst everyone has different reactions to things, there are some general signs that your frequency is weak:

- Numbness of face (particularly when using a mobile phone)

- Headaches

- Excessive or unusual tiredness

- Weakness in muscles

- More frequent illness (weakened immunity)

- Depression

- Sleep problems

- Change in appetite or weight

- Skin breakouts

- Lack of concentration

- Short temper/loss of sense of humour

Once you are aware of your energy, you can forget the labels of illness. I've noticed that as soon as we label how we feel as being a disease or a condition, it makes it much easier for our body to give in. Don't tune in to the frequency of illness – simply focus on how you feel. As you track your energy, you will notice over time where your weaknesses are, so that you can pick up on any imbalances as soon as they happen.

When you open your channels of awareness, you will really start to notice how your energy changes. I wonder if you've ever wanted a new car and as soon as you decide that you want that particular model, you see it everywhere. For any woman who's ever been pregnant, you start to see pregnant women on every corner. We start to tune in to the things that we're thinking about and shift to a different frequency. If you decide to focus on being ill or on being afraid, you will attract to you things that make your illness or your fear worse. But you can also choose to tune your energy in to a vibration that attracts positive emotions and good health.

2. Learn the Art of Healing Through Creativity

Some of the most common ways of coping with emotions are also the most destructive. By using alcohol or drugs to numb their emotions, many people find short-lived comfort, but they are also gambling with their health. Surely there must be a natural way to cope – a way that we can channel our emotions and energy together?

I'm a great advocate of self-expression so the second thing that I think is critical for maintaining energy is creativity – but don't worry if you're not a natural artist. We can express our creativity in many ways: through reading, writing, cooking, flower arranging, gardening, embroidery, sewing, knitting, decorating, tinkering with cars, sculpting, singing or painting – basically through any hobby that we enjoy. One of the ways in which I express myself is by painting.

My mother had a fairly artistic nature, although she didn't have much time to nurture it, given our busy family life. I remember winning a watercolour competition when I was in my early teens, and I went on to exhibit my work in my later school years. Now I favour oil paints and I always paint on large canvases – about a metre and a half high by a metre across. I need this much space to channel, and I like the sheer impact of the space. But I'm not the only one with talent. My brothers both have artistic flair too: Momo paints as a hobby, and Brano chooses to channel his gift into his career as an architect. So I suppose you could say we're all fairly 'arty'.

A lot of artists paint from what they see – interpreting objects and people around them. I paint in a different way. I don't paint still life and I don't paint things that I see in my imagination. My ideas come from a place much deeper inside me and it's hard to put into words. I channel what I feel in the moment that I'm painting. I sense what's happening inside and around me, and this energy comes out on the canvas. I know when I'm ready to paint. I start to see colours and I feel bubbles of excitement rising inside me. I wait for the right evening because I always paint through the night, when I can be alone and at peace. I sense the energy. I anticipate the moment when my energy has built up so much that I have to release it. There is always a reason why I paint: for me, art isn't a hobby – it's a need.

My art only ever has a positive intention. I will often paint when I feel imbalanced or upset, and I counteract the confusion with the powerful, calming energy of my gift. I often paint angels, and the first time I painted them I was having a really rough time: my country was poisoned by war, and I was fighting my own battle in a personal relationship. I was on the way out of this turbulence, and I needed a surge of energy to propel me, to heal me.

One of my most significant paintings maps out my life. At some level I knew that it was time for me to gain clarity about where I was going, and the picture contains images of my son, my mother's death, the arrival of a significant partner and a chessboard, to symbolize the decisions of life. The painting is bursting with vibrant energy and every time I look at it I'm in awe of my journey.

I don't know how a painting will look when it's finished, so I'm usually in suspense about what I'm going to paint next. Like turning the pages of a book and unravelling the story, every stroke of the knife reveals a surprise. It's like watching an epic movie and I revel in every single minute. I feel supported, energized and just plain fantastic – I feel great just writing about it! Afterwards I feel comforted and at peace with the world. I look at the painting and it feels like it's someone else's work, as if an external force has guided me. I know when it's the right time to paint, rather like I knew when it was time to write this book. I just had to do it.

People tell me that they look at my paintings and feel strong sensations. They don't need to understand my interpretations, they don't even need to look at the detail – they just need to gaze, to feel and to lose themselves in the energy. By painting, I transform energy from my heart out through my hands, in a similar way to when I'm treating someone. I can feel the frequency as I create the picture, and my mind and body float on the wave of energy.

When we do something that nourishes us, we get lost in the activity and it returns us to our natural frequency. One of the areas where this is very clear is with music. Sound has a powerful effect on us both physically and emotionally, and it can stimulate or depress our immune system, blood pressure and mood. Each sound has its own frequency, and if the frequency resonates with us, it can restore our cells and organs to a state of balance. So when we listen to or make music, the vibrations of the notes move through us and affect our energy. Sound has been used as therapy for centuries in Egypt, Tibet, India, Greece, Italy, Japan and China. Thousands of years ago the Chinese believed that music could do everything from transforming someone's character to restoring the fertility of the soil.

Most of us practise our own version of music therapy. We instinctually make or seek out sound to express our emotions. As babies, our first method of expression is through our voice; mothers sing to soothe their children; when we're depressed, we play or make our favourite music to lift us out of our gloom; and when we're celebrating, we play upbeat music to enhance the mood. I remember singing to my son when he was a baby to soothe him, and I also played music all the time so he'd get used to noise. I think Bojan also found the noise comforting as a lot of babies panic that if they can't hear anything, they must be alone, so by hearing the music, he always knew there was someone nearby.

I guess it must have had quite an impact on him, as he's now a musician – but his tastes have changed from the lullabies I used to sing him!

Music mirrors our mental, emotional and energetic state. One of the best examples of this is heavy-metal music. Many teenagers listen to it as it mimics the strong emotions of puberty – frustration, lack of control and confusion. At that age it's cool to have that energy, but as we mature, our music taste changes. There's nothing right or wrong about taste; it's just a matter of maturity and development and is a part of the learning process that shows how the mind and body are changing.

I play the piano and sometimes compose music to express myself. The year war broke out at home I remember dreaming that I was on a huge stage and in the middle of the stage was a beautiful white concert piano. The auditorium was full, and the audience was waiting for me to play. I kept thinking, 'I can't play, but I can't leave either. Everybody is waiting for me.' I started to play the most fantastic music. It sounded like waves and water cascading – it was quite extraordinary. When I woke up, I tried to remember the piece and could only manage to recreate about a third of the depth and complexity. I still play that music but have never managed to play it as I did in that dream; but it doesn't matter. You don't have to be a professional musician to enjoy music, which is a good job! I can't imagine a world without music.

We all need to find our own creative outlet, even if we believe we're not the creative type. You may not be good enough to turn a hobby into a profession, but you can channel your energy and help to balance your health. When you allow yourself to be creative, you will slow down and see things more clearly. Whether you like to write, paint, make music, sing or dance, chances are, you will express different parts of your personality when you do those things. By sharing areas of ourselves that are normally private, we have the chance to see things that we may not have noticed before. Some people find that art often reflects their emotional state and that through painting or writing they can release the problem, but not many people are aware of this.

> I know for a fact and from personal experience that healing works on many levels. When I first met Seka my paintings were very dark. Months earlier I finished the series 'Torsos and Objects in Space', and most of the figures in those pictures had no heads. When I showed my catalogue to Seka, she commented on the headless figures and said that she thought it might be because I had been beheaded in a past life. I didn't think any more about it, but a few months later and after more healing sessions, I became aware of a subtle change in my work. My figures now had heads, and the mood in the pictures had become lighter and happier. I was using a brighter colour palette, and I developed a sense of freedom in the way I worked. This wasn't something I'd consciously changed – it was just a side effect of the emotional clearing out.
>
> Over the years Seka cleared me of so much blocked emotional and physical energy that I started to become a clear channel for healing energy myself. I am now an accredited healer with the College of Psychic Studies and subsequently I started to develop as a psychic and a medium. For that alone, for all her strong healing energy and for our great friendship, I will be forever grateful.
>
> Marie-Paule

Writing and reading are also great releases. As you've been reading this book, my words have been affecting your energy. The meaning and frequency will have caused a shift in your vibration and you probably haven't even realized it. Sometimes we can find ourselves unable to put a book down – the plot or the characters may draw us in, but we are also attracted to the energy that we experience through the words and frequency of the writer.

The power of healing is not limited to hands-on treatments. We can heal through any hobby or activity that we find relaxing and absorbing. Energy is diverse and works in many different dimensions, and when we explore these dimensions, we channel not only to ourselves but also to other people. We can choose to keep ourselves in a good state by feeding on positive vibrations. Remember that you don't have to be a professional – just create something that feels right to you and go for it. Trust that you can do it and when you work in this way, you'll create something that nourishes you.

3. Keep Moving

The third thing that's vital for strong energy is activity. Some people use exercise to release their blocks with walking or swimming or more vigorous sports like running or skiing. Gentler exercise forms like tai chi, chi gung or yoga can be really helpful in balancing energy. The body is designed to move, and as long as you choose the right exercise for you, it will help to keep the energy channels in the body flowing. By helping to move energy, these exercises keep the body well nourished and in equilibrium.

Anyone who is well enough should take some form of exercise to help maintain their energy levels, and nine times out of ten people also claim that it helps them to heal. The only time that exercise is contraindicated is in cases of serious illness, for example if someone has problems with their liver, gall bladder or pancreas. We can't guarantee that doing activity will be safe, and it's always important that someone follows their doctor's advice. But in the case of most of my patients, I recommend some form of exercise.

Swimming is particularly good because you have to keep moving in water or else you sink. I know that may sound funny, but this is an important consideration if I'm treating someone who's been inactive for a long time. We can all limit ourselves with our minds, so by giving people an exercise that means they *have* to move, it helps to override any mental barrier they may have. Cycling outdoors is also a great choice because the body has to balance and you also have to concentrate on the road, so there's less room to think about the effort or distance covered. Again, it's important to distract from any negative thoughts like 'How much further?', 'I'm tired' or 'I can't do this.' However, whilst in theory some activities may be better than others, the key thing is to find something you enjoy doing.

The things I love the most are walking and running in the open air, and I'm lucky to live near Hampstead Heath so I can get a regular fix of the outdoors. I also find it very relaxing to take a walk in the middle of my working day to clear my head and at the weekend my husband, Don, and I will often spend hours walking around the beautiful open spaces of North London, stopping for a cup of coffee to watch the world go by.

Body and Mind

There is a difference between what I call 'mechanical' exercise and 'mindful' exercise. If you're distracted from what your body's doing, you won't get as much benefit as if you really put your attention into your actions. Our mind controls our energy, so when you feel your muscles working, you can make them work harder and you'll become even more tuned in to your energy changes. When I'm running, if I start to feel tired, I think about a professional runner and how they use their body. I imagine that my muscles can work in the same way and my body starts to react more powerfully. This has kept me going many a time when I felt as if I was running on empty. I also control my breathing by counting my breaths. By focusing my attention on getting as much oxygen as possible into my body, I can't think about how far I have to go, how many minutes I've been going for or the fact that my lungs hurt.

Take the time to listen to your body. You may want to take off your headphones or put down your magazine and pay attention to what's happening to you. Set yourself goals and keep your attention on that goal. By using your mind and body like this, you'll want to achieve more and you'll also enjoy the process. You'll soon become more aware of how your body changes when you exercise and how your movements affect your energy – both when you're healthy and when you're unwell. You'll start to know your body at a whole new level and you'll find that you want to take better care of it.

Moderation

It's important to keep activity in balance. Some people spend too much time being inactive and stagnating, and others are overactive and can't sit still, which can be equally damaging. Because my job is sedentary, I need to do quite vigorous exercise to counteract the mental work I do all day. When I am treating patients, I have to be in a meditative state to rise above my emotions and my conscious mind. I do this so that I don't question the information I get and so I just trust whatever I pick up on. But as I'm in this state, my metabolism slows down and my physical body becomes flat, so I have to balance myself with the opposite force of activity. If I didn't balance myself with exercise, my physical energy could easily drop even lower. On the other hand, if I was running around all the time, that would be as dangerous for my energy. Like balancing a seesaw or a set of scales, we have to make sure we regularly bring ourselves back to a neutral point.

When I was trekking in the Himalayas, I couldn't understand why our guide would insist we do yoga after a long hike. Some days we'd walked for eight hours, so I thought we deserved a rest after that! But I could see afterwards how the yoga smoothed out my energy after the rigours of the climb. By doing a contrasting activity, the body found its equilibrium and felt even more energized.

The key to being active is being able to keep your activity moderate. There's a fine line between doing enough exercise to get all the health benefits and doing so much that your body has no time to rest. But it's hard to be prescriptive about how much to do because everybody is different. As you become more aware of your own frequency, you'll be able to notice the difference between getting the balance just right, doing too little so your energy stagnates and doing so much that you burn out. Some people are naturally lethargic and can happily sit still for hours, so they need less exercise to balance them. Other people, usually those who are typical Type A personalities (characteristically impatient and on edge), cannot function without regular bouts of challenging exercise. You may think you fall into a particular category, but I'd encourage you to experiment because you may be out of touch with what you really need. When you pay attention to your energy, you'll start to notice how your digestion and metabolism are affected by your activity and you'll recognize how much you need to do to keep your energy in check. As you become more in control of your frequency, you'll learn what's best for you and your health will definitely improve.

Little and Often

The final thing I want to say about exercise is that it's best if you build a routine. Our brains like routine – not one that's so rigid that you become a slave to it but one that helps our brain to accept the habit. You don't need to exercise every day, but by doing something every other day or three times a week, you will put in place a way of regularly managing your energy and you'll also be more likely to keep it up.

If you don't have time to set aside specifically for exercise, you can still be active. Find short slots in the day when you can do something. When you're in the car, you can do a bottom-clenching exercise; if you have a desk job, you can find a reason to get up and move every half an hour – perhaps to get a glass of water or to go to the loo; try getting off the bus or train one stop earlier and walk for ten minutes; use your breaks to get some fresh air; and take the stairs whenever you can. It's such an easy excuse to say, 'I don't have the time,' but if your health is important to you, you'll make the time.

4. Eat for Energy

One further area that I've found to be important in self-healing is food. We need the energy in food to stay alive and healthy, and what we eat has a profound effect on the way we feel – physically and mentally. Everything we eat eventually becomes a part of us, so it makes sense that the quality of what we eat will determine how healthy we are. If the body is not properly fed, it cannot help itself in the healing process, but when we eat well and keep hydrated, our energy increases, which makes it easier for us to deal with any challenges. Although I don't follow or recommend any particular programme, I've found that there are some general guidelines that underlie any successful balanced diet.

Liquids

What we drink is important, and I always recommend that my patients drink a lot of pure bottled or filtered water. Given that our bodies are made of up to 80 per cent water, it's critical that we stay hydrated to allow our metabolic functions to take place – and that includes healing. Drinking water is one of the simplest changes we can make to improve our health.

Another liquid that can greatly affect our energy is alcohol. I ask my patients to avoid alcohol on the days that I treat them. The healing process can speed up the metabolism, so alcohol will get into the bloodstream much faster, which puts unnecessary strain on the body. There's no point in giving the body more work to do, and it's best that the body just focuses on healing.

Sugar

It's best to avoid eating sugars and refined and processed carbohydrates that contain a lot of sugar, such as confectionery, white bread, pasta and rice, potatoes and excessive alcohol. We only ever need two teaspoons of sugar in our bloodstream at any one time (and that's to fuel our brain), so when we eat any more than this in one go, we overload our system. When we eat too much sugar, our pancreas has to work overtime and tends to release too much insulin to cope with the sugary rush. If we become addicted to sugar and keep mistreating our pancreas in this way, it will start to malfunction and will no longer regulate our blood sugar properly. Because the body isn't designed to deal with such overloads, we can end up with a whole host of health problems: diabetes, frequent headaches or migraines, tooth decay, poor immunity, yeast overgrowth (and digestive problems), skin breakouts, lack of concentration, mood swings and, of course, obesity.

Caffeine has a similar effect on the pancreas, so make sure you have sugar and caffeine in moderation. The money you save by not buying these foods can go towards healthier foods. Good choices to replace these foods are: wholemeal bread and pasta, brown rice, oats, rye and other wholegrains, fruit and vegetables.

Nutrients

We need vitamins and minerals to stay alive because every process in our body needs nutrients. If we fill up on junk foods, almost all of which contain no nutrients, we become depleted in vital vitamins, and this has a depressing effect on our energy. Our frequency starts to shift and we find that we can't remember how it feels to be healthy and full of vitality. However, I don't like to recommend vitamin and mineral supplements for prolonged periods of time. If you've been eating a poor diet or if you've been ill for a while, then I'd suggest taking a supplement for two to three weeks only to help the body recognize the frequency of these vitamins. The body has to remember how to absorb these nutrients from food so that once your body gets used to their energy, it will be able to absorb them naturally and you can stop taking the supplements.

I sometimes recommend a special juice recipe to my patients, which I find is particularly good for boosting the immune system, and it doesn't cost much to make. Take one kilo each of beets, apples, carrots and honey (yes, that's a lot of honey!), juice everything and have half a cup of the mixture first thing each morning until it's all gone. I find this works wonders.

The best way to get the right nutrients is to eat a variety of foods. Choose foods of different colours and fresh foods that are in season: that way, you're more likely to give the body what it really needs. Remember that good health comes from good food and what you eat today will be a part of your body tomorrow.

Good Fats

It's also important for our body to receive regular doses of essential omega fats. These play a critical role in many metabolic functions, including digestion, hormone production, liver cleansing and healing. Without these oils we can't expect our body to work well at all. These oils are so vital to health that I'd recommend you take a reputable supplement each day if you can afford it. If you're going to spend money on one supplement, I'd suggest an essential oil, as it's the most important thing for your health.

You can ask your local health food shop which oils they stock, and they will be able to suggest one for you.

You can also get good doses of these essential fats by regularly eating nuts, seeds, avocados and oily fish, like salmon, mackerel and sardines. For a long time these oils were overlooked because we tended to believe that eating fat would make us fat and unhealthy. That may be the case with saturated animal fats, but apart from actually helping you to burn body fat, these special oils will only do you good.

Be Gentle

I'd only suggest eating a lot of raw food if you have a strong digestive system, as most people literally can't stomach a high-content raw-food diet. Steamed vegetables are gentler on the body, and steaming still retains the goodness of vegetables. I also don't see any harm in eating meat, although I would say that, in my experience, women tend to need less meat after the menopause. This is something that most women realize anyway when they start to pay attention to how their body feels when they eat.

Something else that can help with digestion is live yoghurt. I always recommend that people who need antibiotics eat live yoghurt or take a supplement of the active culture acidophilus to help their digestive system. Live yoghurt is cheap to buy and also provides us with a natural source of protein, calcium and carbohydrate.

Slow Down

If we all ate small amounts and we ate them slowly, so that our energy was calm, we'd notice how different foods affected our energy and we wouldn't need any advice at all on what to eat and what to avoid. Our body is intuitive and can tell us what we need. It's a bit like having your own nutritionist with you all the time.

All you need to do is start to pay attention to what you put into your body and how it makes you feel. Most people will feel low and lethargic after eating a fatty, sugary meal, but they either think that's a normal and acceptable way of feeling or they don't realize that they can feel any better. On the other hand, I don't know many people who feel bad after eating a piece of grilled fish and fresh vegetables. The answer is inside us – we just have to listen to it.

Weight

One of the most common areas where people have issues with food is with their weight. Being overweight is more common than being underweight, but both situations are detrimental for our energy. When strain is put on our skeleton and our organs, our frequency shifts and this can knock our whole body out of kilter – not many people realize quite how much our weight affects the rest of our health. I always encourage people to take a long-term view of weight loss or weight gain. If we put ourselves under pressure to change our body overnight, we can become thrown off track by the pressure. Any change to our diet is best seen as a life change.

Moderation – Again!

Most of us have weaknesses – after all, food is also to be enjoyed. I love a little bit of dark chocolate and the occasional wood-fired pizza, and I truly believe that it's fine to eat foods like these in moderation. The key thing is to respect your body, which means not eating these foods all the time. What we put into our body has a significant impact on our health. There's a lot to be said for enjoying the nourishment of good food, but I think that the healthiest diet is one that is balanced.

Over the years I've noticed an increase in the number of people who put themselves under pressure to be healthy. I know this sounds a bit odd, but striving for the perfect state of health is not always the healthiest way to live. We all know that if we want to live a long, energetic life we need to eat well, stay active and respect our bodies. But some people can take this too far and become obsessed, doing themselves more harm than good. The mind can block our energy, so if we're continually uptight about having the perfect body, we can become even unhealthier.

One of my patients had been suffering from food allergies for two years. She came to see me claiming to be allergic to not only the usual suspects like wheat, dairy products, yeast, sugar and caffeine but also to so many other food groups, and her diet consisted of one liquid supplement. She got no enjoyment from food and was in a perpetual state of anxiety. Her fear of food had made her ill. As soon as I started treating her, I knew that she had destroyed her immune system. The doctor who'd diagnosed her allergies had made her obsession worse. These were some foods that didn't suit her particularly well, but she wasn't allergic to them all. By believing that she had food allergies, she had created a hostile environment in her body and it had begun to react in an allergic way. She had shifted her body's natural frequency so much that it eventually did find it hard to digest food. She had created the situation.

I told this woman to focus on relaxation and rest – which she thought was mad! I also told her that she could eat whatever she wanted. I have to admit that I was surprised when she did as I suggested, and it took less than a week for her body to accept the foods that it had rejected for so long. Her disease had been caused by her own mind – her own dis-ease with food.

I was brought up to have a healthy relationship with food, and I realize now that my parents gave us a very balanced diet. We ate together as a family and we started every meal with a clear vegetable soup – not because we were aware of getting our five portions or because we wanted to fill up but just because that's what everyone did. We didn't eat too much chocolate because

Mum told us that it was constipating, but we weren't hung up on the junk-food issue, and we also ate a lot of natural live yoghurt, which helped our digestive system – we hadn't heard of wheat allergies or dairy intolerance!

For the most part I recommend a fresh, natural diet, avoiding sugary, processed and fatty foods. I know that some health foods can be expensive, but if you buy the best that you can afford and change your priorities so that you spend money on nutritious food rather than on junk, you'll be able to add in some new, healthier elements to your diet. If you are easily tempted, you may want to start by clearing out your kitchen and stopping buying anything that you know isn't good for you. Many people only snack on sugary, fatty treats because they're in front of them, so turn your attention to buying natural food and do what you know is right for your body.

5. Learn Energy Breathing

You already have a lot of information on how to start healing yourself, but one of the most fundamental things, to teach you is how to use your breath to move your energy. When I mention breathing to people, they often look slightly confused. We breathe automatically and the great thing is that we don't have to think about it. Anyone can breathe, that's for certain: if we didn't we'd be dead! But it's more challenging to combine your breath and energy at the same time.

What is Energy Breathing?

We have energy in every part of our body, and what I usually deal with when I treat someone are blocks of energy and areas where energy flow is weak. So from feeling energy move inside people, I have learned that there are certain energy paths in the body. What energy breathing does is help you to move your energy along those paths on your own, so that you can keep your frequency strong and in balance. This has both mental and physical benefits. If you spend a lot of time thinking or concentrating, this breathing will help to ground you and connect you to your body. And if you're always on the run, the stillness of the exercise will help to keep you in equilibrium. Remember, your body and mind are connected, and energy breathing is the perfect exercise to bring the two elements closer together.

The path of our breath is through our nose and/or mouth and down into our lungs, where the oxygen gets passed into the bloodstream to be transported around the body. Energy breathing is different. While you're doing the exercises that come later in this section, I want you to forget where oxygen goes and just think of where your energy is moving. To help you with this, there is a visual element to the exercises.

You can't see energy, but you can imagine that you can see it by pretending that it's like air moving through your body. Even though we know this isn't true, it gives you something familiar to visualize and focus on. You can just shift your focus and intention from where the energy is to where you want it to go, and this can have great therapeutic benefits. When we're in pain or we know that an area or organ is sick, we can use our breath and our focus to move the energy through that area, helping to release any blocks of negative energy.

In the main exercises, I usually suggest that you breathe up through the body so that the energy comes into you through the base of your spine, or root chakra, and leaves the body through the crown of the head. In some circumstances, you can send your energy in whatever direction you feel is right for you. You'll see what I mean in a moment, when you have a go.

General Guidelines

Before you start, here are a few guidelines:

- Sit or lie down in a quiet and comfortable place where you can be at peace for a few minutes. Make sure that you won't be disturbed at all. I find that a sitting position is best because you're more likely to stay awake.

- When you breathe in, draw the breath down into your diaphragm (just below your ribcage). This helps you to breathe as deeply as possible and to avoid shallow breaths.

- You may choose to listen to music – it's your choice. If you do, make sure it has a gentle rhythm and one that matches the pace of slow breathing.

- You will probably find it easiest to do these exercises with your eyes shut. This will help you to block out any distractions and focus on what's happening inside your body.

- Adopt an open position with your arms and legs uncrossed. This keeps your energy channels open.

- When you have been breathing and visualizing energy for a few minutes, you may start to feel energized and even perhaps a little buzzy! This is due in part to the increase in oxygen in the brain but is also due to the movement of your energy. So after you have finished, spend a few moments relaxing and bring your attention to your surroundings. Energy breathing can be very powerful, and a few minutes of it can cause you to feel light-headed, if you're not used to it. When you're ready, get up slowly and steadily.

How to Focus on the Present

It's simple to describe how to energy breathe, but the hard thing is achieving a state of relaxation deep enough to allow you to do it well. You have to start by training your mind to focus, and once you can focus well, your body and mind will automatically relax – and then you'll be ready to breathe with your energy. Our brain is like a muscle, and if we want a muscle to be strong and effective, we have to train it. So rather than going straight into energy breathing, I always start people off with two exercises to get their mind in top form. The key thing, after all, is to practise by repeating the exercises.

1. Find a piece of music that is played by two instruments, for example a violin and a piano. Play the piece through and just appreciate the music.

2. Second time around I want you to listen only to the violin. I find that the easiest way to do this is to imagine that the violin is someone you really care about – a child, relative, partner or a close friend. By connecting the violin with your emotions and your thoughts, the piano starts to disappear.

This exercise requires such concentration that it forces the analytical part of the mind to switch off, and by shutting down this potentially distracting mindset, the mind becomes calm and focused. You may wonder what this has to do with healing yourself. This exercise takes a lot of concentration and focus, and when our mind is fully engaged in an activity, we can't think about anything else. There is literally no space left in the conscious part of our brain to think about what we're going to have for dinner or what we have to do at work tomorrow. This helps to free the mind, which begins the process of relaxation. You will also find that by having to pick out one instrument from the whole piece, it will become easier to pay attention to subtle signs and feelings in your body. There is so much going on in our body at any time that to heal ourselves, we have to learn to block out the 'background music' and read only the important messages.

Now, for the second exercise on focus.

1. Draw a picture of two concentric circles – the inner one should be green, and the outer one pink.

2. Put the picture a metre or so away from you and look at it for a few moments.

3. When you've done that, close your eyes. You will see in your mind a reversed image of the circles, like a photo negative – the inner circle will be pink, and the outer one will be green – that's just how the mind will see the picture. What you have to do is switch the image back to the original, with the green circle inside the pink one.

4. Spend a few minutes switching between the two images in your mind.

Do you always see the positive in something, or do you tend to see only problems and worries? What this exercise does is teach people to reverse the way they see things, like comparing a photograph with its negative. I wonder if you've ever been feeling great when someone told you, 'Oh, you look terrible!' If you've ever been in a situation like this, you'll know how easy it is to turn an emotion on its head – and sadly, it usually happens this way around, with good feelings being replaced by negative ones. It's such a useful skill to be able to alter your viewpoint, as our energy can get damaged when we focus on the negative elements of a situation and fail to see the positive. If you have the ability to turn around your feelings, then you can make sure that you always protect yourself from the negative by seeing the upside. This isn't easy to do, but because it takes a lot of concentration, it can be very relaxing. People usually find that they're focusing so hard on changing the colour of the circle that they don't have any headspace left to think of what's worrying them!

The way in which we look at a situation will determine how that situation affects us and also how it affects our health. If we want to maintain our health and heal ourselves, we must learn to stand back and see things in a different way. For example, if you always react in the same way to a situation but you're not happy with that reaction, say you always get stressed when you have to give a presentation, this exercise will teach you how to see this situation in a different light, so that you let go of the damaging feeling of stress. Most of us acknowledge that dis-ease can be a precursor to ill health, but we can learn how to minimize those uncomfortable feelings by changing our perceptions, and this exercise is a great starting point.

How to Focus on the Future

Once you've started to tune your mind, a very powerful exercise to help you focus is to imagine an event in the future and train your mind to be there as if it were now. I do this whenever I have a goal that I really want to achieve. By imagining I've already done it, I make it much easier for my body and mind to get there.

1. Find a quiet place to sit where you won't be disturbed for at least five minutes.

2. Think of something that you want to happen in the future – make sure it's a positive image and something that you really want.

3. Imagine you're in that situation now. Use all of your senses to

experience what you'll see and hear and how you'll feel once you've reached your goal. Stay in the future experience for a few minutes or until you start to feel your energy change. You may feel strong or excited, as if you know this will really happen.

4. When you feel ready, bring your attention back to now and take a few moments to orient yourself before you move.

When you do this exercise, you prepare yourself for what you want. When it does actually happen in the future, you'll be ready to deal with it and accept it. You can repeat this exercise every day, and it will help you to create and attract that energy into your life.

You can do all three of these exercises a few times. Once you're comfortable that you have control over your mind, you can start to read your body and maintain your energy. What also happens as you become really good at focusing and controlling your mind is that you will find it easier to achieve a deep state of relaxation.

Preparation Exercise

Once you have learned how to focus the mind, by doing the two initial exercises and the exercise on focusing on the future, I ask people to do a preparation exercise. This exercise takes a few moments. It helps you to connect with all the parts of your body and is simply a precursor to full body breathing.

- Start by breathing deeply through your nose for a few moments.

- Turn your full attention to your body by focusing on each part in turn. Start with your toes. Put your attention into your toes and notice how they feel. They may start to tingle with energy or they may feel heavy with relaxation. Wait until you have felt your awareness fully in your toes before you move on.

- Then turn your attention in the same way to your ankles. Once you feel your awareness there, move on to your calves, and knees and so on, working your way upwards through each part of the body.

- Once your breathing is deep and steady, you can do a specific exercise.

Full Body Breathing

This is the main energy breathing exercise that I teach people. It's fantastic for general self-healing – mental and physical – and it's something I always do in my seminars because it's the perfect time to teach people, when I have them in front of me. I always enjoy doing this myself because it feels so good, and you'll see how powerful it is.

As with all energy breathing exercises, this exercise is a form of meditation. As a rule, I'm not a great believer in set methods for meditation because I find it such a personal thing, but this exercise is one meditation that I find very valuable. Some people find that they slip into a meditative state when they listen to music, when they walk, when they cook, paint or swim: it's a case of finding something that helps you to switch off and relax, and that doesn't have to mean sitting still in a quiet room. In my opinion, meditation is about being in control of your mind, your energy and your soul. We can all benefit from switching off once in a while, so that we're not always on standby, ready to jump into action, and this is a great way to do it. It's a way of bringing together breathing and self-healing, and whilst it seems very simple, it can have a significant impact on your health.

- Start to breathe through your nose as deeply and smoothly as you can.

- Once you feel relaxed, as you breathe in, imagine energy entering the base of your spine, the root chakra.

- With your intention, send the energy up the spine.

- As you breathe out the first time, let the energy leave your body through the crown of the head. Repeat this cycle a few times. This is the main path of energy through the body, and it brings the Earth's energy into the body through the spinal cord.

- On the next cycle of breaths, move energy up from the base of the spine as before, but let the energy leave the body through the centre of your forehead, just above your eyes. This area is known as the third eye.

- On the next cycle, send the energy out through the throat. Repeat this a few times, remembering to breathe deeply throughout.

- Move on to let energy out through the heart chakra (located on the sternum). At each stage, breathe deeply through any discomfort or resistance you might feel.

- Start the next cycle as before, but this time the energy exits the body through the solar plexus, just below the ribcage.

- The last cycle of breaths sends the energy out through the sacral chakra, which is just below your navel.

- Once you have completed all six cycles, spend a few moments centring yourself before you move.

This exercise moves the energy around the main energy channels and helps to clear the body out, whilst giving the mind a break. It's safe for everyone to do.

Once you are comfortable with this, you can focus on areas in the body where you know you need most attention, and you can imagine the path that the energy will take to clear out these areas. I have given three very different examples here to show you how versatile energy breathing is, but these exercises can be adapted for all parts of the body.

Energy Breathing for the Solar Plexus

The solar plexus is the main chakra in the body. This exercise is great for helping with any chest-related problems, such as palpitations, chest pain, breathing difficulties and lack of oxygen to the lungs. It's also good for relieving stress, particularly if you hold your tension in your upper body. It helps to clear one of the body's main energy channels, so can benefit anyone.

- Imagine that as you breathe in, you're pulling energy into your chest area through the solar plexus.

- As you breathe out, send that energy through your chest and out through the middle of your back.

- Keep repeating this pattern of breathing and visualizing for a few minutes. Any pain you feel may increase during the first few breaths, as the negative energy resists, but as you move the energy a few more times, the pain eases. Focus all your attention on your chest area and become aware of what you feel there.

- Repeat this until you feel your body settle down and take a few moments to centre yourself.

Energy Breathing for the Ears

This is good for earache, problems with balance and inner-ear conditions.

- As you breathe in, imagine energy entering your body through the base of your spine.

- With your intention, move the energy up your spine and into your head.

- As you continue to breathe, send the energy out through both ears at the same time and imagine it leaving the body.

- Continue this cycle, breathing deeply through any discomfort you might feel.

- When you are ready, take a few moments to centre yourself.

Energy Breathing for the Ovaries

This is a good exercise to do if you are having any menstrual or fertility problems.

- As before, start by putting your attention into your body and get into a rhythm of deep breathing.

- Imagine energy entering your body through your ovaries.

- As you continue to breathe, direct the energy up the body and out through the crown of the head. Send the energy right out of the body.

- Keep bringing fresh energy in through the ovaries and move the energy through any resistance you may feel.

- When you have completed several cycles, bring yourself back to your centre.

We often ignore the parts of our body that need attention. You can see that these exercises make you face up to any area that needs help. It helps to have a process to follow to help unblock any negative energy because by engaging your mind in moving the energy, you won't think about the problem itself. The beauty of this exercise is its simplicity, and although you need to focus, you'll find it gets easier with practice.

When you first begin to do energy breathing, you may find that it takes up to half an hour to prepare and then do the exercises, but as you get used to it, you will find it much easier to get into a relaxed state and you will be able to complete the whole process in about twenty minutes. It's a very relaxing thing to do before you go to bed, or you can take a break in the middle of the day, but you don't have to do it every day. If you can start by doing it once at the weekend and once during the week, you will notice a big difference. You will find that once the meditative state comes easily to you, you will be able to do this breathing pretty much anywhere.

By breathing more consciously, we immediately pay more attention to our body and our energy. Once you get really good at controlling the movement of your energy, you will sense exactly what your body needs. With practice, you will be able to direct your energy to wherever it's needed – it's all about how well you can control the movement with your mind. I recommend you begin with the exercises at the start of the chapter to focus your mind. When these exercises become comfortable, you can move on to the energy breathing exercises that will keep your frequency clear and strong.

I know that breathing has been recognized as a significant factor in well-being for a long time. In some cultures people have been using their breath and intention in this way for centuries. The fact that so many people across the world have been doing this for many years proves how vital breath is to health. Energy breathing is one of the most important elements of self-healing, and it's something that I have practised myself for years.

6. Know Your Boundaries

We're all human and part of our nature is that we are fallible. We have weaknesses, we have 'down' times, and we feel emotions – that's what makes life colourful. But a normal healthy life can become plagued by the drive to push ourselves beyond what our body wants to do.

I learned the hard way what my boundaries were: I found what I could and couldn't do by pushing myself to extremes. That's one way of finding balance, but a much safer and more sensible way to do this is to recognize in the first place that you have limitations. I had to experiment through trial and error because I knew nothing about my gift, but for most of you, you will be able to sense, by tracking your energy, what you can and can't do.

We all have things that we naturally do well, and when each of us works with these talents we find that we fit together like a jigsaw. No particular talent stands out as any more important than another – they're all just different. Anyone who has ever had an unsuitable job will be able to relate to this. Whether you took a job because you needed the money, or you made a mistake and thought you were doing the right thing, you'll remember what it feels like to try to fit in to a role that simply wasn't suited to you. I'd guess that you weren't happy or healthy, and the sad thing is that some people put up with this because they think it's normal! This is not normal – or natural. Life will feel natural when you discover what you need rather than what you want – and that includes your job, your relationships and your lifestyle. This also applies to healing, and you should learn what you're capable of.

Everyone can heal to a lesser or greater degree. I'd encourage you all to use this power but learn what your limitations are. Begin by working on yourself, because you'll only do a good job on others when your energy is strong. Notice how your energy affects others when you're around them. We send out energy to other people all the time through giving advice and love and by sharing our time and our thoughts. All of these things are forms of healing, so make sure that what you send out attracts the right people to you and keeps your energy strong. If you wish to experiment more, work on minor ailments first, like headaches or stomachaches. Be honest with yourself as to how you feel during and after treatments and accept that there is nothing wrong with having boundaries.

I have learned that I need a certain amount of pressure and drive to keep up my energy levels. The obligation I have to treat people means that I can't be ill very often, so because I don't want to let other people down, I find that my energy is strong almost all of the time. I can sense when I'm taking this too far, and I make time for myself.

Once you become aware of your boundaries, you will have to learn to say no. Your health comes first, even if part of your life involves caring for others. You cannot look after other people unless you are strong and healthy, so accept that when you say no to someone else, you're actually saying yes to yourself. Remember that when we work at our optimal level, we find that we are happy, balanced and successful, but if we push ourselves too hard, we can often damage our energy. Be clear on who you are and what you can do.

7. Learn to Protect Yourself

Every time we connect to another person, physically or mentally, we exchange energy. We connect to people without being aware of it, so because most of us spend a lot of time around other people, we are all at risk of becoming drained. It's important that we learn how to rid ourselves of negative energy and that we protect ourselves as best we can.

I was born a healer and that's why I am able to work at a consistently high level *and* maintain my own health. Once I knew what I was doing, it was easy for me to protect myself, and I have a high level of natural resistance. But we're all vulnerable – and this can be hard to admit. I would advise anyone who is nurturing a healing gift to be very aware of their own energy. We all get drained from time to time but you're much more susceptible to low energy if you're constantly giving it away.

Please manage your own energy first and foremost and recognize when you need to recharge: none of us can effectively help others unless we look after ourselves. I learned to protect myself so that I could lead a normal life. I got into the routine of closing down my energy channels to stop myself from collapsing and getting ill. Although I now close down my channels automatically, I still avoid situations that I know will drain me. We all have to be as strong as we can and remain as detached as possible from other people's emotions. If you do this, it doesn't make you heartless – it means that you'll keep yourself strong.

Knowledge is protection. What you will have learned throughout this book is that the more information you have about energy and the things that affect it, the more chance you have of keeping yourself healthy. You can protect your health by being aware of external energies and by increasing your sensitivity.

8. Avoid Electromagnetic Pollution and Geopathic Stress

As you know from reading Chapter 7, two of the greatest drains on our energy are electromagnetic pollution, which is a by-product of modern technology, and naturally occurring geopathic stress. We can't get rid of these so what we can do is become aware of them, so that we can reduce their effects. Here are some simple tips for you to follow.

Tips to Avoid Electromagnetic Pollution

- Use your mobile phone only when you have to or for quick calls; otherwise use a landline.

- Protect yourself from your computer with a protective screen that you can buy from any computer supplies shop.

- Avoid sitting with electric cables under your chair or desk.

- Where possible, avoid spending any time near power stations.

- Remove electrical equipment from the bedroom, including radio-alarm clocks, hairdryers, televisions, electric blankets, mobile phones, computers and cordless digital telephone bases.

- Set up your digital telephone base and wireless Internet connection in a part of the house where you don't spend much time.

- Turn off your broadband when you're not using it and don't get a wireless network unless you really have to.

- If you can, switch to an analogue phone – you can buy cordless ones.

- Remove electrical toys, for example train sets, from your children's bedrooms.

- Do not sleep on a metal-spring mattress.

- Do not sleep on magnetic pillows or mattresses.

- Only use baby monitors when you absolutely have to.

Some Common Symptoms of Geopathic Stress that you Should be Aware of:

- You have a serious illness.

- Your illness isn't responding to appropriate treatment.

- You've tried a number of different therapies – conventional and complementary – without success.

- Your symptoms clear up or improve when you are away from home, for example on holiday.

- You became ill shortly after moving house.

- Your home has never felt comfortable and you felt ill at ease as soon as you moved in.

- You wake up feeling groggy in the mornings, even when you've had enough sleep.

Some Signs of Geopathic Stress in the Home:

- There is mould in the house.

- There is a lot of lichen or moss growing on the roof, walls, or lawn. (These plants thrive in areas of geopathic stress.)

- You may have a problem with ants, wasps or bees, as they are attracted to these energies.

- Cracks in walls, driveways, paving slabs and roads may be a sign that your home is on a geological fault line.

- There are trees that have split in two or that have large knobbly or strange growths. If the branches look as if they're trying to get out of the way of something, they probably are.

- Certain plants like to grow in areas of geopathic stress, particularly oak trees, firs, elderberry, peach, cherry trees and mistletoe.

- Your close neighbours are in poor health.

- There are springs or wells nearby.

- Previous occupants of the house were ill.

- Animals are sensitive to geopathic stress. Horses, dogs, cows, sheep, pigs and mice would not willingly sit over areas of geopathic stress, so if the dog has a favourite spot in your house, it's safe! On the contrary, cats are attracted to geopathic stress so avoid sleeping or sitting for long periods anywhere that your cat likes to settle.

If you experience any of the above symptoms, try moving your bed or sleeping in another room and see how you feel. This should, however, only be a short-term measure until you can seek professional advice. You can contact the British Society of Dowsers (www.britishdowsers.org), or I personally recommend Alf Riggs (www.alfredriggs.com).

9. Manage Your Emotions

We can't avoid having emotions, but we can reduce the ones that pose a threat to our health. Whilst it's natural and healthy to feel negative emotions from time to time – such as anger, frustration, sadness, grief and guilt – what isn't healthy is an excessive amount of any of these. All of these negative emotions depress our natural energy and leave us weak and open to illness, but the worst emotion of all is fear.

We can all relate to fear, whether it is fear of heights, public speaking, spiders, rejection, loneliness or failure. There are so many fears to choose from that everyone has at least a handful! What you need to understand is that fear causes the greatest damage to our health and is the root of many other negative emotions. You need to learn to see your fears for what they really are, so that you can protect yourself.

One of the best things you can do is face your fears and laugh at them. After all, many of the things we are afraid of are fears that we have made up in our heads. Laughter mitigates the effect of stress hormones in the body and also stimulates the immune system. Laughing is like having a dose of magic medicine, so find as many reasons to laugh as you can!

One thing I have noticed from treating many cases of prostate cancer is that these patients are often full with anger and other negative emotions because of problems that they've had in their personal relationships. There is a close connection in particular between the guilt that comes from having an affair and prostate cancer. But what I find surprising is that even when their body is suffering because of what they've done, some of these people find it hard to acknowledge that what they did was wrong.

In order to change something for the better, we have to admit that there's something wrong in the first place. Although it may seem like an obvious thing to say, I'm forever amazed by how many people find it hard to acknowledge that they've made a mistake. We can't be expected to get everything right – we are only human – but I believe that as long as we always act with integrity and honesty, we can correct anything.

If our energy is blocked or drained, life doesn't flow, so it's often not the mistakes themselves that count – it's how we deal with them that matters. What all of my advice will do is help you to increase your self-awareness of your behaviour and how it affects your energy. There's nothing wrong in admitting that maybe things are not quite the way you'd like them to be. Once you recognize that, you can change your life to improve your energy and your health.

10. Keep Growing

From my experience, one of the best things we can do to keep our energy strong is to keep challenging ourselves. If we settle for too long, we stagnate. Our bodies and our minds love to be stimulated, and it's very energizing and uplifting to do new things. When we do something for the first time, we get a real sense of achievement – like a buzz – and that buzz is our energy vibrating at a powerful frequency. Although it may seem hard, the best time to push ourselves is when we least feel like it.

I was faced with one of my greatest challenges many years ago when I was on holiday in the Himalayas. I had been in Tibet for a few days and was amazed by the energy of the place. It's so vast and powerful, and I had really started to feel like I was part of the environment. I had never experienced energy quite like that. One day I went with a group to climb one of the Himalayan peaks. Half the group was in their twenties, so I was one of the more 'mature' members. Most people had been training for the climb, but I had only made the decision the day before to do it. I guess I must have got carried away by the energy around me, as part of me knew that I wasn't physically fit enough. The last section of the climb was at high altitude, and people started to drop out and stay with one of the guides. My legs were numb, my breathing was really laboured, and my heard was palpitating. My body was telling me to stop so I sat down to pull myself together.

If I'd been sensible, I would have called it a day and given in to the fact that I wasn't fit enough, but I didn't. I gave myself a stiff talking to! I had to reach the peak. I don't know why, but I just felt that it was something I had to do. I knew that it would take me at least another four hours, and I thought, 'If I die here, then it's meant to be.' I don't often do things like this, but I just made a decision to push myself. As soon as I made the decision to get on with it, my head cleared, and I just got going. When I got to the top, it was like I was dreaming. I was breathless, not because of the climb but because of the view. I felt on top of the world.

I came down ahead of everyone else. I had gone from being at the back of the group to leading the way. I had no pain, I breathed comfortably, and I felt fantastic! This was the first time I had really experienced the true power of my mind, and it made me realize that if I could do it, then so could everyone else.

When we can't make up our mind about something, we waste a lot of energy dithering and deliberating. But once we make a decision and commit ourselves, we find that all of the energy that we were wasting on being indecisive gets channelled into the task in hand. When we focus our intention and energy, we can be strong beyond all belief.

I was ill from 1982 to 1989, with many ups and downs culminating in three years basically in or on my bed. I used to have ambition, determination, a successful career and a general tendency to burn the candle at both ends. Obviously, all this came to an end when I was ill, and I had to give up everything and retreat to my parents' home to be cared for. The frustration I felt was in proportion to my previous headstrong, active, 'go-get' character.

My misery came to an end when, after trying many other treatments to no avail, I had two weeks of therapy with Seka. Within those two weeks I regained my energy and strength and was able to begin building my life again.

It's now seven years after seeing Seka. I have been working full-time for the last three years with practically no sick leave. I play squash, hike, cycle and swim. I'm currently studying for a Master's degree and have also married and recently had a baby.

In short, I am now fully recovered and busy. However, I learned my lesson and am now very careful to look after my health, to eat well, sleep well and to live in the present, rather than constantly running after future goals. I am very thankful that I had the opportunity to meet Seka, and I now appreciate every moment of my life and re-found health.

J.

The Final Word

Healing may seem complicated because, in the West, it's a concept that is far removed from our everyday lives, but that doesn't mean that it doesn't work. There are plenty of things that are integral to our lives of which we have no understanding, and we just take them for granted. It would help if more scientists were open to researching the field, as for some people, testimonials and healthy survivors aren't proof enough: they want to see scientific evidence. I'm also open to further research, as I'm fascinated to find out more and I feel strongly about letting people know about the real power of healing. When it comes to healing, it's as if we're conditioned to disbelieve, which I find rather sad. Remember that some of the world's greatest discoveries were mocked and rejected for decades before they were proven and widely accepted.

We know that we can heal ourselves because we've all experienced it first-hand. Whether it was a mouth ulcer, a cut, a cold or a broken bone, we have all witnessed our body regenerating. As a child, I remember the scabs on my knees and elbows that soon disappeared, giving way to new skin, and this was probably my first memory of healing. You will be familiar with these notions of healing, and I hope you can now also see that you can prevent symptoms and illnesses from appearing in the first place and that this preventative self-care is also a valuable element of self-healing. Our bodies have intelligence and capabilities beyond our wildest imagination, and all we have to do is tap into this body wisdom by becoming aware of our energy shifts. We are made of energy, so when we learn about Bio-Energy, we are also learning how to take care of ourselves.

Our bodies are designed to regenerate, and our cells are continually dying and being reborn; so we are healing all the time. But despite this knowledge, healing still provokes very mixed reactions. Some people are firm believers, some are adamant disbelievers, and others have no idea what to believe! I think that this range of responses is partly due to the fact that healing encompasses a wide range of practices. When a mother places her hand on her child to calm them, it soothes and brings comfort. When a friend gives another a hug of support, it relieves some of the pain. And when we put up our feet after a heavy day and sip a cup of tea, we feel calmed and revived. When we eat well and exercise we are regenerating and rebalancing our bodies. When we lose ourselves in a good book or become engrossed in a movie, we are also healing ourselves. Healing happens when we sleep, rest, laugh or share a problem because all of these things change our energy Every single thing we do, think and feel impacts on our health.

When I first started healing, I was overwhelmed by the dramatic changes I could help people achieve. I was amazed by how someone could be seriously ill one day and healthy the next. But as the years went on and I discovered more about how our energy behaves, I realized that the less spectacular, invisible shifts are just as important. One tiny crack left untended widens into a bigger fracture, which becomes a rupture. By managing your own energy, you can patch up the cracks and pre-empt more serious illness. Whether I'm helping cure someone of eczema or whether you're ridding yourself of a negative emotion, it's all healing.

Many people either believe healing to be a complicated and spooky phenomenon or they just don't believe it at all. Up until now there has been very limited information on how Bio-Energy works and how we can all bring it into our lives. I have talked to you about living intuitively, and my intuition told me that it was time to write. I'd thought about writing before, and I'd even been approached by writers and publishers, but I knew that I wasn't ready to share myself and the world wasn't ready to listen. Now that we are more open to preventative natural medicine and the idea of healing, the time is ripe. Initially, I was confused by my gift and I thought that healing must be beyond human comprehension. What I've come to realize through years of experience is that the answer to good health and self-healing lies in making a few simple choices in life.

When I treat someone, it's vital that they carry on their own healing work. Ideally, I don't want to see people come back time and time again with serious conditions. I recommend having regular treatments to boost energy, but I always hope that my patients take away enough knowledge to teach themselves how to maintain and balance their own energy.

Hopefully, this book will have given you a new insight and passion for healing. Just by reading it, I'm sure you've started to pay more attention to how your energy is affected by people, places, thoughts, emotions and situations, and I have faith that everything will become clearer to you as you start to experiment. You have the basic tools to use your own gift – you may not be able to heal others, but I believe you have the power to heal yourself. Your energy is continually shifting, and the sooner you can sense these subtleties, the sooner you will feel and see improvements in your health.

I'd encourage you to take in this information and start to make small changes every day. It doesn't take much extra time or effort to take care of yourself. I find that when I've learned something new, the best thing I can do is put it into practice straight away. So, if you haven't already started, it's time to become aware of your own energy and begin healing yourself.

If you are interested in finding out more about Seka's work or if you would like to attend one of her seminars, please visit www.sekanikolic.com.

Visit **www.panmacmillan.com** to read more about all our books and to buy them. You will also find features, author interviews and news of any author events, and you can sign up for e-newsletters so that you're always first to hear about our new releases.

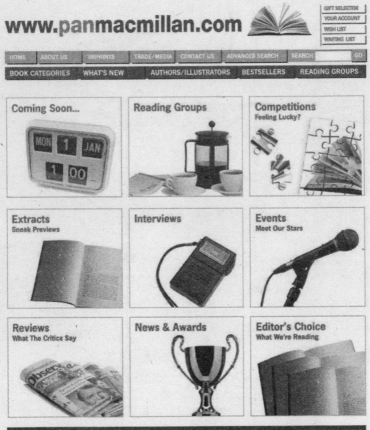